F🍴RK YOUR DIET

Michele Neil-Sherwood, DO
& Mark Sherwood, ND

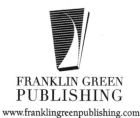

FRANKLIN GREEN
PUBLISHING
www.franklingreenpublishing.com

"Do you want to feel better and be able to enjoy life to its fullest? If so then his book is for you. It is full of practical and effective strategies that can change your future."

**Dr. Bob Harrison,
"America's Increase Authority"**

"This book is an arsenal of must-have information for combating the root of sickness and maintaining wellness! As a frequent traveler with a loaded schedule, which revolves around ministry and television production, I have found it difficult to maintain consistency with my health and weight management. It is with heartfelt gratitude, that I offer a big thank you to Doctors Mark and Michele for writing this book! It is easy to understand and full of practical applications that enable you to live the wellness lifestyle in any given situation. I highly recommend it for everyone!"

**Brenda Crouch
Author, Speaker,
Singer, TV Co-Host**

"Drs. Mark and Michele's book and blogs have changed my life, way of thinking, and the way I personally practice medicine. Their multifaceted approach treats the whole person: mind, body and soul. Their fearlessness and passion for people is inspiring. They have an incredible way of encouraging and motivating change and I love the way they challenge our thinking about wellness. I have used their principles to teach my patients how to become healthier. They are a blessing and Godsend to the medical community."

Monica Woodall, D.O.

"Functional medicine is the future, and Drs. Mark and Michele bring a modern understanding based on personal history and years of training to help patients recognize cardiovascular risk early – and do something about it. Using the latest cardiovascular markers of inflammation as part of their integrated approach to wellness, the authors provide patients with knowledge and tools that are easy to understand and implement, so they can live well and live longer."

**Dr. Marc S. Penn, M.D., Ph.D., FACC,
Co-Founder and Chief Medical Officer,
Cleveland HeartLab**

"This book is a must read! In all my years of traveling, I realize how easy it is to lose sight of a wellness lifestyle in the constant pace of deadlines and changing time zones. A big thank you to Dr's Mark and Michele for this easy to read, practical, yet articulate, guideline encouraging every reader to live the wellness life in any circumstance with utmost quality. I highly recommend it for everyone."

**Paul Crouch Jr.
American Television Broadcaster,
Film & Video Producer,
Speaker & TV Co-Host**

"I hope this book inspires you as much as it did me. It is a must for anyone wanting to experience the benefits of a healthy life."

**United States Senator,
James M. Inhofe**

An important note to the reader:

This book is not intended as a substitute for the medical advice of physicians. Readers should regularly consult a physician in matters relating to health and particularly with respect to any symptoms that may require diagnosis or medical attention. Do not make changes to your diet, exercise, or intake of prescription medications without consulting your physician.

The names of patients and other details in the stories have been changed to protect the privacy of our patients.

This book is dedicated to all of our wonderful patients around the world who have inspired us, as well as our family and friends who support us as we all carry the torch for true wellness.

Contents

Acknowledgments

WE WANT TO SAY A GIGANTIC "THANK YOU" TO ALL OF THE many contributors to the book, as well as those who are key to the inspiration behind it. As we began this journey of writing and researching this book, we began to think about all those who have formed our foundation of support.

To our parents and families, thank you for your love and support. I know we brought you challenges at times, but you continued to put a roof over our heads and clothes on our backs.

To our friends who often refer to us as the "food police," we know your jests were always in good humor, and we appreciate you for encouraging us.

To Mike Loomis, dude, without your help, this book would not be what it is. Your diligence and work ethic was masterful. As a member of our team, you were a star. To Lee Gessner, we all need publishers, right? Thank you for putting up with our questions, emails, and comments. Together, we created a winner that will transform lives.

To our support staff, what would we do without you? Becky, Fawn, Jackie, Jill, Jennifer, Onnah, Emily, Felicia, Sheila, Kade, Beth, Melissa—we love each of you dearly and are honored to be a part of your lives. (I, Mark, am a hormone expert, as you can see, since we have all women in the office. Therefore, I understand estrogen dominance and truly don't mind it a bit.)

To our many medical mentors, thank you for your leadership.

To our readers, we thank you for your support in this cause called wellness. Our world is better and more healthy because of you. We are thrilled you carry this torch together with us. Together we are bigger and brighter.

Thank you for helping us spread the true wellness movement and change the world, one life at a time.

Foreword

Dr. Kellyann Petrucci

IN OUR PURSUIT OF WELLNESS, WE TYPICALLY FOCUS ON exercise and nutrition—but there is a much deeper issue we need to address. Often, our inner hurts and wounds trigger self-destructive behaviors, ranging from a sedentary lifestyle to poor nutrition and emotional eating. They can also cause fatigue, a "wellness debt," emotional instability, and chronic illness.

These roots of disease, known by the acronym FRAUDS (fear, resentment, anger, unforgiveness, disappointment, and shame), can grow into mighty forests that obscure our view of who we are as individuals and cause us deep suffering. To be truly healthy, we need to face, deal with, and eradicate these roots.

Drs. Mark and Michele totally nail it in this book. With practical advice and directives, coupled with inspirational success stories, they show you how to free yourself from FRAUDS and achieve the true wellness you deserve. Their message is inspiring and empowering, and I truly believe that this book will transform millions of lives. I know I'm excited—I hope you are too!

Dr. Kellyann Petrucci
Author of NYT bestseller
Dr. Kellyann's Bone Broth Diet,
and host of the PBS special
"21 Days to a Slimmer and Younger You"

HEALTHY FROM THE INSIDE OUT

There are many promoted paths to wellness. But only one leads to continual success.

Maybe you've tried one of the many routes that start with exercise and diet. And maybe you've failed—even after temporary success.

We invite you try a different path.

Yes, we care about your physical health. But what we're truly passionate about is helping you find lasting wellness in every area of life.

Our approach might be different than normal. But "normal" is not working. So how about a fresh start? Ready? Set? Let's go!

1

I Was Blind

A few months ago, Michele and I were working out at the gym. I climbed onto an elliptical machine, which is a cross between an exercise bike and a treadmill, and opened the reading app on my phone. A few minutes later, after I began to break a sweat, a gentleman stepped up onto the elliptical next to me and opened an app on his phone. We'd seen each other several times but had never met. He was about forty-five years old and at least that many pounds overweight.

In other words, he looked "normal."

Keep this concept of "normal" in the forefront of your mind as you proceed through this book. Prepare for your preconceived definition of this word to change!

After observing this man pedal on that piece of equipment for just a few minutes, I noticed he was sweating profusely and breathing like a locomotive. With each gasping breath he took, I actually wondered if he was going to need CPR.

At about the same instant, we looked at each other and happened to notice we were both reading the Bible. After some friendly conversation between breaths, I learned his name was

Jerry. He had been trying for some time to shed some weight by showing up at the gym to improve his health. We chatted at length about the health struggles he was having and his desire to lose some weight. The struggles he was having seemed normal for a guy his age.

Conversations like this are not a rare occurrence for Michele and I. People often ask us questions about their health, and we're honored to be asked. But there was something unusual about this talk with Jerry. I could tell he was on the verge—on the verge of failure in his quest for wellness.

First, he had the wrong goal—lose some weight. Now, there's nothing wrong with losing excess weight, but that should not be your primary goal. I know that may shock some of you, but hold tight—you'll understand exactly what we mean very soon. How many times do you see people in the gym year after year and their body composition does not change? They may be exercising more, at a higher intensity, but their true health status and weight/muscle status does not change—they may even accumulate more excess fat. You may have even experienced this yourself!

Second, even though Jerry had shown up to the gym and climbed up on the exercise machine, I could see he was tired—not physically tired, but tired of his weight-loss battle. We've seen this look hundreds of times before. People are always going on a diet, making resolutions to change; yet the root of the problems remain unchanged. Year after year, this approach to health and wellness leaves many exhausted and tired and without hope. This is certainly an area in which we can all relate!

Jerry had lost hope. He continued to work out in spite of his emotional turmoil and inability to change his overall health.

We know this feeling of hopelessness ourselves. Growing up wasn't easy for either of us. We had to dig deep at many different points in time to find the will to carry on. Interestingly, we were both adopted and had challenging upbringings. Self-esteem, eating habits, and health were issues for us both too. We didn't know any better. No one ever taught us—about wellness or about life in general.

We've had to pick ourselves up off the ground over and over. And today, our experiences in having overcome those challenges are what help us guide people out of the roots of sickness and disease and help them put their feet back on the pathway to health. We're able to instill within people an attitude and a lifelong *Quest for Wellness* (our other best-selling book). So get ready to have the best life ever as we take a moment to unpack our stories. Also, don't forget about Jerry—his story will blow you away!

Mark's Childhood

I (Mark) was a frumpy and sometimes chunky kid—a little bit weak and picked on at times. Believe it or not, even today, when I look in the mirror, I see that dumpy, frumpy kid.

Fast forward a few decades. After trying for a couple of years and failing to make it in professional baseball, I became a police officer. During my time in the police department, a horrible tragedy occurred in my life, along with an equally tragic series of observations. This is very hard to communicate, but I want to share it here. When I was thirty-eight, my mother committed suicide, which devastated me in more ways than I even understood at the time. Her encouragement in my life had been so important to me, and to this day I miss her morning calls to say, "I love you."

While working in the police department, I began to observe a very disturbing and concerning pattern. I watched how men and women would join the police department in the best shape of their lives and die in the worst shape of their lives shortly after retirement. And they weren't living very long in age. The life expectancy of a retired male police officer was sixty-six years old. This fact shocked me, because I was on track to be one of the people who made this average expectancy so low. During my time in this career, I saw people die, I observed the chaotic potential of society, and I looked into the eyes of evil. I guess all these experiences were used to bring me some unique perspective.

One day, it hit me like a ton of bricks. What we're doing, and how we're living, isn't working. In fact, it's killing us. This had affected my family as well as the men and women with whom I was serving. What was going on? This really began my tireless pursuit for answers. I was dead set on trying to understand what really makes mankind tick and what drives both good and bad decisions with resulting positive and/or negative consequences.

Using the same methods and insights as we're outlining in this book, I took hold of my health and decided to make it a life mission to help others. I've been so fortunate and blessed, even in those hard and devastating times, to tour the world with a group strength-performers and motivational speakers whose mission was to offer motivation and hope.

Michele's Childhood

I (Michele) grew up feeling like I was a parent to my parents. This statement isn't meant to imply that my adoptive parents didn't love me or to make them appear like bad people. My father suffered a tragic accident and was disabled when I was twelve years old. A physical accident sometimes hinders more than just the physical. The emotional and spiritual state of a human being can be injured by physical injury. He really never recovered.

He later became riddled with disease and, as time passed, became morbidly obese. His lifestyle lacked any demonstration of what health should look like. Later, my mother became progressively disabled after she retired. With their health issues, I found myself trying to play rescue and help remedy the situation any way I could.

Through the years, I saw them both try, and fail, to get their health under control. They tried every fad diet without success. I watched them try numerous vitamin pill regimens and read health magazines and books, all to no avail. It grieved me that they couldn't make lasting progress in the right direction dealing with the totality of "wellness" in their lives, and my witness was one of watching them suffer. Their suffering was in most areas of the four- dimensional person (physical, emotional, intellectual, and spiritual).

As a result, I took on a "compulsive health nut" approach. I loved my parents but was horrified at the sickness, disease, and obesity issues that afflicted their lives. In my heart of hearts, I felt compelled to help them find a better way. I sought information in an effort not to be like them and in hopes that I might help them with my studies and learning processes.

I remember reading one of my father's go-to health books, written by Adelle Davis. I incorporated a lot of her principles into my life and began taking a handful of nutraceuticals that were supposed to increase energy and strength and help with weight loss. I further read all kinds of health magazines myself and found myself delving into exercise. I climbed the ranks of judo quickly to achieve a brown belt.

After my sophomore year in high school, my family found itself in the state of Oklahoma. After a job relocation, my mother began working as a nurse practitioner. She was the sole provider for our family. She was smart beyond her time and excelled in academics.

I was heartbroken having to leave my roots. I lost friends, I left my paper route and babysitting jobs, and I left behind my martial arts community and my first love: music. I played eight instruments by the time I was in the ninth grade and had hopes of being a songwriter and music major. Obviously, our move south was not a move I wanted to make.

My high school years were disastrous, as I worked three jobs to help support my family. I worked so much that I almost flunked out of high school. I found a new martial art, Tae Kwon Do. I climbed the ranks quickly and in eleven months received my black belt. I set my eyes on the Olympics, with a dream to be an Olympian when Tae Kwon Do had its debut as a spectator sport.

My mother's job did not last long and left her without work. My family moved back to Minnesota, but I stayed in Oklahoma to pursue my dreams of Olympic glory in Tae Kwon Do (which came to an abrupt end after a left knee injury) and pursuit of a career in massage therapy.

Because of my lack of finances, I was forced to live in my car for several months until I built up enough paying massage clients to afford an apartment. By the early1990s, I was earning just enough money on a regular basis to rent an apartment. For the first six months, I had no furniture and lived by candlelight to save on expenses. With no furniture, I slept on the floor, and after about eight months bought myself a futon that gave some simple creature comfort and a cushion from the hard floor.

My massage therapy career did take me on many traveling journeys to study with some of the greatest healers, health experts, and wellness gurus. I finished a degree in naturopathic medicine in 1995. Then, after a massage client spoke into my life after the completion of my naturopathic degree, I found myself on the medical path.

The road through medical school was indeed an adventurous one. My passion to help people was on a steady increase. I felt in my heart of hearts that medical school was the ticket to truly help people get well. I not only wanted to be in the best health personally, but I wanted that for all the people who would come to me for care. Yes, I met with adversity, but the drive to do better, live better, and be better are and were at the core of my being.

Diet or Live It

As you can see, we both had plenty of opportunities to quit. However, we simply couldn't. Our drive is really fueled from our past experiences of overcoming. We won't quit, and we want you to be infected with that attitude as well.

Our society has more knowledge regarding personal well-being than ever before, yet we're more unhealthy than ever before. The numbers of people afflicted with inflammation, weight issues, metabolic syndrome, and diabetes is rising. If we have all this information at our disposal, what's the disconnect?

I (Michele) began my journey helping people improve their heath as a massage therapist, went into naturopathic medicine, and eventually became an osteopathic doctor. With every new level of expertise and tools, I was still frustrated with the overall health results for most people.

Information isn't the answer to health. And medicine isn't the answer to getting well.

When I started as a resident, there were five medications for type 2 diabetes; today, there are at least thirty. Type 2 diabetes is on the rise and obesity is approaching 50 percent of the US population by the year 2030, according to recent studies.

About 75 percent of our health care costs are spent on conditions resulting from obesity. Cancer, diabetes, heart conditions, joint problems, and musculoskeletal issues all have a close relationship with lifestyle. Poor nutrition and lack of exercise (or improper exercise) leads the chronic inflammation trend. By the way, chronic inflammation is at the root of all chronic sickness and disease.

Diets don't work. Over-exercising doesn't work, and you can't out-supplement a lifestyle riddled with poor lifestyle choices. Even the best medical professionals can't override unhealthy choices. Even God will not override the consequences of our repeatedly poor choices. An example of this would be continuing to speed, get repeated citations, and always expect God to pay the fine. This, in actuality, would be a misuse of the concept of grace. Additionally, medication can mask the root cause by managing blood pressure, blood sugars, and other disease states, but their help in eradication of disease requires that the person with the problem take some serious action.

How do I know this? Because I tried. When I (Michele) was working for a large medical enterprise that pushed doctors to see thirty, forty, or even fifty patients per day, I became exhausted and patient care was short-circuited. Sadly, this is normal in today's society, and I had a hard time remembering people by name. Working at such a pace, one hardly has time to focus on a patient's lifestyle and what has made him or her sick in the first place. You're on a time clock to get to the next patient.

After a few years of this demanding schedule, most doctors (just like me) become exhausted too. With just a few minutes of time spent with each patient, doctors can't really help many people get to the root of their problem. The very people they wanted to help when they chose to become a medical practitioner are suffering. Their true hearts for healing are not able to be expressed when they have to follow an algorithm to quickly shuttle the patient out the door. These algorithms never address lifestyle. Listen, we aren't talking about the lifesaving emergency events when the decisions have to be made fast, such as an emergency appendectomy or the surgery required to reattach a severed limb; we're talking about the ability to address having a high quality of life. As you can see, there's a disconnect between mainstream medicine and true health care.

When you have about five minutes with each patient, your ability to really hear a person's story, understand the person, and come up with an assessment and plan, as well as educate, is extremely limited. For most of us, it's virtually impossible. But what we *can* do quickly is use a prescription pad. This provides a solution for the urgent problem but doesn't get to the root cause of why the problem is there. I had just enough time to look at the chart, know what I was treating, and decide what drug to prescribe or what special study to order for the patient. Sure this method helped in the moment, but was I really affecting long-term change in my patients' lives?

Something wasn't right. This is where so many clinicians and practitioners find themselves. They went into medicine to bring healing. They find themselves working at a pace that is equal to, or more hypervigilant than, medical school. Once out of school, they're carrying hundreds of thousands of dollars in medical school debt, buying their first homes, and raising families. To meet the demands on their personal lives, they get a job in an established medical system. Once there, these young doctors must follow the rules of the system and abide by what insurance companies tell them to do.

The system puts people on the hamster wheel and keeps them from personalizing medicine for their patients.

Health Care or Sick Care?

Unfortunately, we've all been governed by a system that's taken its toll on us. "Health care" is not health care at all. It's "sick care" management.

Pharmaceutical companies are growing, large medical systems are growing, and insurance companies are growing. What's wrong with that? Just one thing: people are less and less healthy.

We believe the system needs to be flipped—instead of rewarding practices that see the most patients per hour, why not reward physicians who actually keep their patients well? This would change culture and improve the lives of countless people.

Can you imagine a world where health was truly valued and was the center of attention? Can you imagine the economic upturn? Can you imagine how the supply of what we now demand (processed food and drugs) would change? Trust us, if you don't buy it, they won't make it. We all need to get wise to what is really happening and why.

Yes, we could write an entire book on this subject. But we want you to know our motivation. There are wonderful, caring people on both sides of the system. We're simply pointing out that the system is broken.

We're thankful for medical breakthroughs, including medications, but the ultimate goal should not be medicine. Our mission is to eliminate unnecessary medicines and eliminate self-imposed, choice-driven diseases. The ultimate goal is wellness.

We also want you to know that the book you're reading isn't your average "feel better" message. While we're challenging the system, we're also going to challenge you.

Faith and Action

The questions our society currently asks about health and wellness need to be questioned. As a matter of fact, normality needs to be rigorously questioned.

People go on diets and try something new for three months, fail, and then go back to the same old bad habits. Many people don't have a clear understanding of how our bodies are naturally designed to keep us healthy and how we're meant to enjoy nutritional wellness.

Instead of asking, "How do I lose twenty pounds?" why aren't we asking, "How do I maintain my optimal weight?"

Instead of asking, "What new medicine should I take?" why not ask, "Am I eating the right foods?"

We need to understand that lifestyle is the key to long-term wellness. Food is medicine. As Hippocrates stated, "Food is thy medicine and medicine is thy food." He was a man far ahead of his time. If you give the body what it needs, it will heal itself. These healing components come from the air we breathe, the water we drink, and the vital nutrients we feed our bodies.

Where Do We Start?

A man of faith named Daniel lived around 600 BC. He and his countrymen were forced from their homes and taken captive to live and serve in a foreign land. Everything about this new culture was different, including the food.

While imprisoned there, Daniel saw a connection between their native diet and the fact that he and three of his fellow Israelites were not feeling well. He proposed an experiment to his captors. They agreed. Talk about favor! Can you imagine negotiating with your own kidnappers and getting them to actually listen to you? Amazingly, Daniel's proposal involved changing their food intake for ten days. Instead of eating the traditional diet of the country, said to be a lot of meats, breads, and wine, Daniel proposed a diet of fruits and vegetables. After ten days (yes, only ten days), everyone saw the positive results. This first God-designed clinical case study showed such positive benefits that everyone in not only the prison, but in the entire kingdom, took notice. The king even promoted Daniel and his colleagues, not only because of their physical health, but because of the wisdom they displayed as well as their appearance. *Yes,* they even looked better. Nutrition had changed their foundational state of health.

So what happened next? Everyone went back on their old diet, right? Wrong. The king not only let the new diet continue but promoted it as well. The kingdom was now going to go Daniel's way! You see, Daniel had enough belief in and knowledge of how to care for himself that he influenced others. Many don't continue on a course even though they know it's right and it works because those close to them (friends, family, or coworkers) are not following along. Daniel was resolved. He had made up his mind and transformed his heart to believe in the cause. Wow! We all need to take a pause right now and learn this powerful lesson from Daniel.

Unfortunately, the pattern so many of us have followed goes like this: go on a diet, lose weight, achieve your "goal," and then go right back to your old ways of living. The standard American diet fails us every time. We end up right back where we started—oftentimes worse. We end up heavier and more inflamed. We end up on more medications. Surely there's not a feeling or sense of well-being that comes with this yo-yo phenomenon. It's more like feelings of tremendous shame, guilt, and self-pity.

There's even a very popular diet called the Daniel Fast. The question is, if this change brings positive results, why is it a temporary change? What are you "fasting" anyway—poor foods that cause inflammation and lead to disease? Really? Are we this naïve and gullible? We have to do better, because we are better than this.

So if we have access to the latest science and the healthiest foods, why are people getting worse? Instead of seeking out the latest fads, why not develop a lifestyle of eating foods that helps us feel better every single day?

The reason why is simply because we don't create a new mindset and a new lifestyle, and because a wellness lifestyle is simply not "normal" in our society. When it comes to health, people who try to live differently are often ridiculed and thought of as odd, just like Daniel was. (But instead of a fiery furnace, we're threatened with a pizza oven and a deep fryer!)

If we offer you a proposal like Daniel and guarantee you would feel better and look better if you followed our plan, would you go for it? All you have to do is work the plan and reap the aforementioned rewards. So why not? What do you have to lose? Really, the question should be what could you stand to gain?

Refresh your memory on the concept of New Year's resolutions. Isn't a resolution a promise you make to yourself? Why do we break these promises to ourselves day after day and year after year? Why do resolutions have to be repeated anyway? If we make a promise to ourselves (and others), let's simply keep our word.

Daniel was consistent in his words—and his actions. And we'll help you with both in this book. All we want you to do right now is resolve to be well and feel better!

I Was Blind

Remember Jerry, the gentleman we met at the gym? Well, he took us up on our proposal. He made an appointment to see us at our clinic and became a patient. As a new patient, he went through a battery of common tests and a full physical examination. Testing included body composition analysis, EKG, full blood panel (including chemistries, lipids, certain vitamins, hormone testing, and inflammatory markers of heart disease). Tests indicated he had active markers for metabolic syndrome, heart disease, hormone dysfunction, and an obese body composition. These were not the results he had expected, as he had been told by his PCP (primary care physician) that he was normal. He had been told he needed to watch his cholesterol, not eat too much sugar, lose a bit of weight, and get a little exercise.

We spent time with Jerry trying to get to the root of his problems. We dug into his lifestyle and began to understand why he was so unhealthy. Putting together his test results, his lifestyle, his past life experience, and the exercise regimens he'd tried, we came up with a new plan for him. He had to make some *big* long-term lifestyle changes. These changes had to occur in order for him to change his life. Stay with us on this subject, and we'll explain to you exactly what's needed to obtain lasting and long-term change in your own life.

Jerry followed all our recommendations and made big changes. Within three months, he lost fifty pounds. This loss came strictly from yellow fat. His body composition measurements improved by 14 percent (he lost 14 percent of his body fat and increased by five pounds of lean muscle tissue), and he looked like a different man. His out of bounds cholesterol and blood sugar levels, and several other inflammatory markers, returned to normal, except one. The one issue that had to be handled to maximize his composition was hormone balance. His hormones had to be replaced. Keep in mind, a thorough evaluation and understanding of his history allowed us to formulate a plan that was individualized just for him.

We both ran into Jerry at the gym recently. "Hey, Jerry, you're looking great! How are you doing?" we asked.

"Can I share something with you?" he asked. We nodded as he continued. "You know, I was blind."

With a puzzled look we asked Jerry, "What do you mean?"

"I thought I was seeing clearly, but I was totally blind. I would see myself in the mirror and think I looked all right. My doctor told me I was normal for my age. I just had to watch my blood sugars, cholesterol, and exercise. I'd look around at everyone else and think, *It's just normal to be this way (a little overweight) and feel this way.* But now, for the first time in my life, I can see."

Jerry realized it was his lifestyle that was at the root of his problem. He had to make radical lifestyle changes in order to bring his life in order. He had no idea how the standard American diet was killing him.

Jerry's entire life changed when he realized that "normal" was killing him.

Do You Want to Be Well?

This sounds like a ridiculous question, doesn't it? While most of us aren't really afraid to die, what we do not enjoy is the process. We don't want to endure the chronic disease and suffering that appears to happen in later years. So, do we really want to do what it takes to be well?

Your desire is the only part of the journey we can't provide. You must bring your own "want to."

Let's be honest. Some people get their identity from being sick. Have you ever asked someone how they were doing and heard, "My arthritis is flaring up," or "My diabetes is being controlled better." Why do we claim these diseases as *mine*?

Medical professionals take an oath that includes a promise to *first do no harm*. But what if a practitioner withholds truth that could be helpful to a patient—isn't that harmful? Consider type 2 diabetes—is it a symptom or is it a disease?

You have to really wonder about this disease. It didn't used to exist, but it's rampant in our affluent country today. We have excessive sweet treats, an overabundance of fast food restaurants, and grocery stores full of non-foods that drive this disease. We'd be negligent not to mention the massive advertising that's used to promote consumption of non-foods that drive these types of conditions. Think about it: athletes and celebrities promote sugary sweets and insulin-elevating products under the guise of health, beauty, wealth, and optimum performance. In reality, the opposite is true.

New patients normally find their way to our practice because they are tired of being sick. They've seen a lot of doctors and still have the same issues. They don't have any guidance, they don't have a plan, but they really want to be well.

If someone has a strong desire to enjoy health, we can put them on the right path. Without desire, all the guidance in the world won't make a difference. So don't waste your time with this book if you don't truly desire an improved quality of life. But if you do, trust us, and be willing to question everything you've been taught about food, medicine, and health.

Question "normal."

Obviously, "normal" isn't working.

The Most Honest Patient We've Ever Seen

You've doubtless filled out forms at your first visit to a doctor's office; our office is no different. One of the questions on our form is, "What is the reason for your visit?"

Before we greet a new patient, we review the form. Most of the time the answers are pretty vague: *don't feel well* or *want to lose weight*.

Ben's form was pretty standard until we read the two-word answer to the question about his visit: *I'm dying.*

We were shocked and went immediately to his exam room, hoping to find him alive! Thankfully, Ben greeted us warmly. He was a nice guy in his early sixties, married, with children and grandchildren. He was also obese and barely fit in the chair. Wondering how to begin the conversation, we asked him to clarify his answer.

"I'm really dying," he said with tears in his eyes.

"What are you dying of?"

"The doctor says I need to lose eighty pounds before they'll operate on me."

Ben's arteries were so clogged up they needed to perform heart surgery (he was in need of a quadruple bypass), but because of his weight and other risk factors (blood pressure, elevated cholesterol, triglycerides, and blood sugar) he was too high of a risk for the operation. He had realized he was dying a few weeks earlier, but in reality the disease had taken root years, even decades, ago.

Then he asked us, "Can you help me?"

We gave an honest answer, which is the same answer we give all our patients. *I am 100 percent confident we can help you, if you'll trust us.* He took us up on our proposal.

He worked the program for approximately one year. One day after he had his appointment with his heart surgeon, we received a message: "Hi, Mark and Michele. I'm almost there, and the doctors are getting ready to schedule my surgery." He had nothing to lose. He made a promise to himself that he'd give the program a 100 percent effort. He didn't waver one bit, and his efforts paid off.

We made sure to be there on the day of his surgery. We prayed for him and gave him careful instructions not to die. After all, he'd come this far; we felt very responsible for him.

Ben had a successful surgery. Not only that, he continued to lose weight and was even able to return to the career he loved: teaching.

During his evolving death process (before he landed in our office), he'd even had to take a leave of absence from his job. As he told us, he was "just too winded and worn out." He thought he was just getting old. In reality, he too was blind to the fact his lifestyle was at the root of his sickness and heart disease.

The standard American diet is normal. Unfortunately, so is diabetes and heart surgery these days. Do you want to be normal?

Healthy from the Inside Out

No matter how hopeless you feel, no matter how much you weigh, no matter the condition of your health, know this: we are here for you. We believe in you and know you can heal your life. It's time to take the blinders off. It might be a little painful at first, just like any acute injury. It hurts at first, but with each passing day, it gets better if you give it the right attention.

If you're like most people, you've tried fad diets. You've tried self-discipline. You're tired of trying harder. What you've found is that *trying* does not work! You have to make the decision to *do*. Our goal is to help you do it right. You'll never have to look back at another failed attempt.

What if we said you were destined to fail with every one of those attempts? Now you should be getting increasingly motivated! Now, what if we said there's a different path—a path that addresses not just your physical body but your mind, emotions, intellect, and heart?

There is. And you're holding the guide right now. Will you trust us?

Helping people take back their health and enjoy their everyday lives is why we wrote this book and why we help people in our practice every day. We get into the trenches with people. We want to get into the trenches with you. We're going to help you get to the root of what's keeping you from enjoying health.

Imagine, just for a moment, becoming a walking billboard of wellness. Yes, you *can* look and feel your best.

We are 100 percent confident we can help you too—if you'll trust us.

2

You in Four-Part Harmony

IF WE'RE GOING TO EXPLORE WHAT WELLNESS REALLY LOOKS like, we must explore what we're made of. And every one of us is made of *PIES.*

No, not the apple, chocolate, or coconut cream kind— although we've seen some XXL T-shirts emblazoned with *Body by Pie.* We're talking about the four-part makeup of every human being:

Physical
Intellectual
Emotional
Spiritual

These four elements are part of our design, and each is designed to be healthy—and in harmony with each other. You simply can't separate them. They all work interdependently— *not* independently.

We all understand the *physical* aspect of our being: our skin, blood, organs, tissues, and cells. If our physical self goes down, the balance of our four-part harmony person will suffer. Make *no* mistake about it. We must care for ourselves physically and never neglect this part of who we are.

We understand the *intellect* because we're reading this book. The very ability to comprehend a written word and have it paint a picture in our mind is fascinating. And the way the neocortex expands as we acquire knowledge is amazing. Just a side note here—keep on learning! The intellect needs consistent exercise too. Some of the greatest leaders in the world practice continual learning.

We can relate to *emotions* because we all get angry, we all get sad, we all laugh. We might not always understand our emotions, but we know how they can affect the other three parts of our being, as well as our relationships. Have you ever had your emotions get out of whack and take you places you never wanted to go, in word, action, or deed? Hey, we've all been there. The emotions need constant work too.

The *spiritual* piece might mean different things to different people, but we believe everyone understands that we're more than a random set of DNA and neutrons. The *heart*, as the Bible often describes this aspect, is the essence of who we are. We all have an intuitive idea of what is right and what is wrong. That's your spirit. Further, we all have a sense inside of us that says *yes* or sometimes *no* or even to *stay* or to *go*. This is the very essence of our identity.

So what does this have to do with wellness and health? Everything.

I thought this was a diet and exercise book.

This book is, and isn't, about exercise and diet. In reality, it's about seeing you live in four-part harmony. This means getting to the root of health issues instead of playing whack-a-mole with symptoms.

All four parts of our being can be healthy or unhealthy. All four can change. All four can work in harmony with each other—or fight each other. And all four parts are interconnected.

We know what food is, and we know that it affects us physically. Your body sees everything you put in your system. Your stomach has to see it, your gut has to see it, and then your liver, kidneys, bloodstream, and brain; your whole system has to deal with it.

But food can affect us emotionally too. If what we eat is toxic—too much alcohol, processed food full of chemicals and sugar, or caffeine—the food alters the gut microbiome to the point where it starts producing toxic neurochemicals that affect emotional health. That's right: our brain becomes what we eat. If we eat "unfood" that lacks nutrition and contains antinutrients, our brain will become unfit and begin to "unthink." Surely we all want our brains and emotions to function properly for the duration of our lives, don't we?

We are what we eat, and we *feel* like what we eat. Additionally, we will become what we eat! You'll know exactly what we mean by this as your journey through this book continues.

Even when we don't get enough vitamin D, an antidepressant, (and the vast majority of people don't), we're more susceptible to being emotionally and mentally depressed.

Think about toxic relationships. If we're around a bunch of negative, destructive influences, we'll become emotionally toxic, which can lead to depression, lethargy, and fatigue. In our practice, we often see patients complaining of physical symptoms that are coming from emotional experiences: physical abuse, emotional abuse, financial issues, and stresses. What you put into your mind creates emotions and can create physical symptoms. Think about a toxic relationship you've had. Did it suck the life out of you? We know it did! Listen, proper pruning isn't just applicable to the garden; it's necessary for forming lasting and solid relationships.

Ever had a stress-related headache? Ever eaten a certain food because of emotions? You have to be thinking now, "I get it, yes . . . wellness isn't just about diet and exercise!" If you are, you are certainly tracking correctly.

When a person is physically sick, he or she usually knows it intellectually. When someone is obese, has high blood pressure, and is on multiple medications, it impacts his or her mind and emotions. Many decide to go on the Internet and start searching for information on how to fix the situation. This journey can be emotionally draining and intellectually confusing. Have you ever experienced information overload? That in itself can drive someone nuts!

Before long you've tried "everything," and none of it has worked, which is upsetting on many levels, including spiritually. Why? Because we were designed to be healthy. And when we don't feel well, we're often less likely to pursue the deeper matters of the heart.

Emotional unrest can cause us not to sleep well. Not sleeping well brings physical, mental, and emotional fatigue, which can lead to weight gain and high blood pressure.

Yes, we're complex beings, with four simple, interconnected parts. This is one reason why making healthy changes can be difficult. Most people will fail to improve their well-being if they don't address all four areas. We've got to understand this as a foundation in order to obtain true wellness.

You Are Not a Body

Who are you? Who do you want to be? How much do you want to weigh?

Most men have to pause and think about their answers. Almost every woman who comes to our clinic has an instant answer to these questions. But in both cases, the answers are usually wrong. You'll understand why shortly.

Then we'll ask, *When you look in the mirror, who do you see?*

If this doesn't prompt a lot of emotion and heartfelt reaction, the next question will be, *Do you like what you see?* The answer is usually no.

At this point, we know the goal is to change the person's vision of himself or herself. We start off with this exercise, and we invite you to join in. Whether you believe in God or not, you'll get the point.

"If God was sitting right here with us, how would He describe you?"

Most people say something like, "I guess I'm a nice person," or "I have some work to do," or "I am kind." We then probe further by asking, "Physically, what does God see when He sees you?"

Many times the answers are, "He sees me as fat," "He sees me as unhealthy," or "He sees me as addicted to sugar."

Listen friends, God doesn't see you as *overweight*. He sees beyond our physical bodies. You have a body, but you are so much more than a set of organs and tissues. He sees you as perfect, with unlimited potential and unfathomable abilities. That's truly what we want you to grasp right now! You are so much more than a body. His love for you is unconditional and not based on performance. Yes, we have responsibility and freedom to choose (we'll help you with that), but you are amazing in every way. Go ahead and say it now, "I'm amazing and perfect in the eyes of God." Say it again and again until it sticks. This is a prerequisite for seeing yourself through the eyes of success rather than failure.

The question to our patient, and the question for you is this: *Then* why *don't you see yourself this way? What went wrong to skew your vision?*

Yes, you do have a body, but you are so much more than that.

And even the true physical you is not the excess coat of fat you might be wearing—it's who's inside that coat! If you're struggling with weight, the real you is struggling to get out of that fat.

Before we can make meaningful and lasting improvement, we must have an accurate image of our physical selves. The next step is to acknowledge this to our intellect.

This Truth Makes Sense

The mind is not the brain. It's important to know the difference. The brain is a physical organ that functions according to a series of chemical reactions that can be triggered by a wide variety of "input" sources—including physical chemicals from food and other substances, as well as emotions and behaviors that trigger neurotransmitters, which govern a wide variety of physical functions.

The *mind* refers to our abilities to think, to reason rationally, to remember, and to make good decisions. There is no anatomical spot called the *mind*. Obviously, we need to be feeding our physical brain with the best nutrients and ideas in order to maximize the function of our mind.

Does the shift in perspective about your physical body, discussed above, make sense to your intellect?

Hopefully so, because physiologically, a person can gain or lose fat and still be the same human being. Therefore, you are *not* the fat you're carrying. It's not part of your intellect, emotion, or spirit—and it doesn't need to be part of your physical being either.

Another truth to acknowledge is that on this journey, and on any new endeavor worth taking, you will struggle and make mistakes. This is a fact, so why shouldn't we be honest about it?

We always tell our patients, "When you fall, get back up and stay engaged with us. We'll always encourage, we'll never pity, but we will say, 'Get up!'" Some people fall down a lot, and that's okay. The only people we can't help are the ones who quit trying. So even if you fall down seven times, get up eight! This is the remedy to never fail. After all, you aren't a born failure; you are a born success.

For some reason, our four-part beings resist change, and any attempt to disrupt "normal" can wreak havoc on your senses. There will be discomfort, there will be pain, emotions will rage, your stomach will grumble. When patients remove certain foods, which we'll discuss, people start to find out who they really are—because they've been covering all four parts of their being with sugar for so long, they've misplaced their identity.

So, with your intellect, prepare. And use your power of imagination to see your destination: wellness, peace, and joy. When you consider the "temptations" you'll face, ask your intellectual self, do I want to feel good for ten minutes during a meal, or do I want to enjoy feeling healthy every waking moment?

Prepare your mind to make the right choices—even when you fall down.

Chocolate or Vanilla?

People don't usually think deeply about what life will be like at age eighty.

Do you want your physical, intellectual, emotional, and spiritual life to be the same at age eighty as it is now?

You may not want to be like your parent or grandparent, but what are you doing to change the outcome? Are your habits taking you down the path you want to go? Of course, we can't choose everything in life, but we have more control than we care to consider. It's like chocolate or vanilla—you choose. Do you want a sick life or a healthy life?

Do you ever think of yourself as the grandparent who sits in a chair and can't get up? You can be that person if you want—that's your choice. Or you can be the grandparent who actually runs after the grandkids and catches them.

For parents and grandparents, the same questions about children apply. *Do you love them?* And the answer is always the same: "Of course I do!"

The generation after you is going to do what you do. Do you want to change your child—and change generations for the better? You can. But you must use the power of your mind to choose.

Prepare your mind. It's worth it.

We must bring all four parts into harmony. Especially those energetic emotions.

The Emotional Dimension

Emotions are very important. They contribute to the way we respond to the physical world around us and to the way we relate to other human beings. They are a part of total health and are meant to be enjoyed.

Our overall health can be greatly impacted by emotions. This happens largely because certain emotions cause stress, which triggers a release of adrenalin into the body. Over time, the body becomes addicted to its own stress hormones, even though the release of cortisol into the bloodstream can have very damaging effects.

Among the emotions that trigger adrenalin and the stress-hormone effects of cortisol are anger, deep sorrow, weeping, hatred, and prejudice. In sharp contrast are emotions that trigger endorphins and are generally helpful to our physical body. Perhaps the foremost of these emotions is joy. Joy, it should be noted, isn't the same as happiness. Happiness is always linked to external circumstances or stimuli. Joy is an abiding emotion deep within a person, often related to hope, love, and our spiritual dimension.

Emotions in Motion Trying to Control Our Lives

Doctors often focus only on the physical aspect of our being. Psychiatrists and psychologists often aim on just our mind. And pastors zero in on our hearts. Meanwhile, emotions are left to themselves and can end up running the show.

The connection between emotions and health, or disease, is surprisingly strong. In the world we live in, our emotions are constantly bombarded.

We've seen health clubs try to entice people to buy memberships with free donuts and pizza. You'd think the irony of the situation would drive people away, but it doesn't. The same is true with retail establishments, and even churches, baiting people with junk food. But why? I know we're touching deep nerves here, but it must be addressed. What are we doing to ourselves and the next generation?

Let's be brutally honest, we use food as bait because it works.

Why does it work? Because most of us have been trained since childhood to connect emotions with food.

Whether it's a birthday party, a church celebration, a funeral, or skinning our knee, for some reason we're offered cookies and ice cream as "comfort" food.

You get your first bicycle. You fall down and scrape your elbow. Mom or dad comes to the rescue, puts on a bandage, and says, "Oh, don't cry. Let's get an ice cream cone, that will make you feel better." Food becomes an emotional band-aid.

When you join your first sports team and have that big win, what happens? Pizza! And after that disappointing loss or blunder on the field? *Let's go get some ice cream—you'll feel better.*

This connection continues into our adult lives. Have a big win at work? Have a devastating day at work? Did a loved one pass away? One answer, often prescribed, is food. In all our emotions, pain, celebration, disappointment, adulation, and grief, we're trained to use food as our friend—to use food to make us feel better. And it might, for a few minutes.

Is it any wonder why food addiction is so hard to break?

Food and Drug

Sugars operate the same neurotransmitter pathways as cocaine. This pathway is known as the reward pathway. The tragedy of this pathway is that it triggers the abusive behavior patterns of addiction. Another tragedy is when we don't find out until our health is destroyed, we are thirty pounds overweight, and we are suffering from the chronic disease that poor choices set aflame years ago.

No one in their right mind would say, "I know you're addicted to cocaine, but here's just one hit for this weekend. It won't hurt you. Just use it in moderation." We wouldn't do that to an alcoholic either: "Let's go have one drink."

Believe it or not, an addiction to food can be just as dangerous, because the emotional connection can run even deeper, from childhood, and because the wrong food can end our lives early. Most aren't afraid to die, it's the suffering that usually ensues before death that we fear. Little do we know, we're contributing to our early death by the horrific ways we've been conditioned to eat. Our emotional selves are often rooted in comfort from food at every occasion.

Imagine saying to a child, "I know that bee sting hurts, but you'll feel better soon. Let's go have some broccoli!" Feel the disconnect? Better yet, feel the connection with reward and food. The brain center becomes patterned at a young age, setting lives up for health disaster.

I (Mark) have experienced this disconnect bringing snacks to kids on a sports team. I brought apples one time, and can you guess how many were eaten? Zero. I was even told, "How dare you bring that kind of food. No one will eat them." You would've thought I'd brought poison apples.

The point is that making a choice to eat healthy foods will run counter to most of society and counter to your emotions.

Food and Love

When a childhood emotional connection with food is based on dictating emotions with health-destroying and toxic foods, is it a crime? This type of eating usually results in obesity, which can lead to disease and early death—even when intentions are good. Let's face it, if we do something to or allow something to be done to a child that's harmful, is that considered child abuse?

We had a patient in our office who struggled with her children eating junk food. When she took them to her mother's house, they were served whatever they wanted, in whatever quantity they wanted. Was the weight problem the child's fault, or did the problem lie in the hands of the one buying, preparing, and providing the food, the source of the problem?

Mothers and grandmothers (or whoever is the household cook) often associate love with food. They express love to their children by making them wonderful breads and sweet treats. After-school treats are sugary in nature and not usually just a piece of fruit or a handful of raw nuts. Holidays commonly consist of three different plates of food and two loaves of bread at one family gathering.

Getting together is a wonderful time to catch up and reminisce, but why is it such an opportunity for gluttony? I (Michele) grew up with a mother who loved to cook. Cooking was one way she loved our family. She had the best recipes, made with what we thought were the "best ingredients." We had fried chicken, meatballs, spaghetti, and loaves of bread, all on one table, and then we had to clean our plates or there was no dessert.

By the time we got to dessert, we were already overfull. In my mother's defense, she always made sure there was a green vegetable served with every meal. What we didn't learn was portion control and understanding of how the most important medical decision we were making every day was and still is at the end of that silver fork. Eating is one thing, but understanding its consequences is another.

The divorce rate in our country is about 50 percent. When parents divorce, most end up having joint custody of the kids. For a variety of factors—and a variety of emotions, including guilt and fear—parents often treat their children to comfort food. As the children get older, and are trained to associate food with love or emotional well-being, the parents become less willing to enforce consistent food guidelines, for fear that the child won't want to visit. Food is often used as "bait" to get children to comply. What are we doing? Besides rotting their teeth, we are influencing their long-term health.

Does all this sound harsh?

This is the first generation in American history when children will be more unhealthy then their parents. It's predicted that one in three children under the age of eighteen right now will be a type 2 diabetic by the time they're forty. This is factual information that can be viewed on the Centers for Disease Control website. All you have to do is look around you and see our youth succumbing to the health-destroying habits driven by emotions. What they don't know is that their choices may cost them their health sooner than later in life.

Nutritionally, the way many are raising their children is a new kind of child abuse. It fits the definition of a crime. If you do something to your child that you know brings them harm, that's a crime.

A New Kind of Child Abuse and Neglect

Child abuse is defined by federal law as:

- "Any recent act or failure to act on the part of a parent or caretaker which results in death, serious physical or emotional harm, sexual abuse or exploitation."
- "An act or failure to act which presents an imminent risk of serious harm."

This definition of child abuse and neglect refers specifically to parents and other caregivers. Child abuse and neglect are certainly serious issues. Obviously, penalties for such acts include imprisonment. When someone thinks of these type of allegations, thoughts go toward physical, sexual, or emotional abuse. But another serious type of abuse is happening every day without being acknowledged.

Let's look at some statistics. Obesity is the leading cause of preventable death in the United States and around the world, according to the Centers for Disease Control. Over two billion people worldwide are overweight, with an estimated 700 million who are obese.

The tragedy of these statistics, which refer to adults, is they affect the future generation as well.

- One in three children are overweight in America.
- Childhood obesity has more than tripled in the last thirty five years.
- There are now more than two million morbidly obese children, above the 99th percentile in bodyweight.
- It's predicted that childhood obesity will have more impact on the life expectancy of children than all childhood cancers combined.
- One in three children born today will have diabetes in their lifetime.
- Obese children six to eight years old are approximately ten times more likely to become obese adults.
- Snacking leads to an additional two hundred calories per day for kids.
- Kids who are overweight or obese may miss more school.
- 70 percent of obese children already have at least one risk factor for heart disease.
- Healthcare costs related to childhood obesity reach $14 billion every year.
- Childhood obesity could reduce life expectancy by five or more years.
- More than one in four people aged seventeen to twenty-four in the United States are now too heavy to

serve in the military, a development that retired military leaders say endangers the nation's national security.

Stress is commonplace for parents. We're all trying to move faster, do more, and accomplish more than humanly possible. As a result, most nutrition for our children comes from fast food and sugar. And in the process, emotional ties to food are being created.

Fast food is full of heavily processed grains; sugary carbohydrate sources; low-quality meat; sugary sauces; low nutrient density; trans-fats; hydrogenated oils; additives; preservatives; red, yellow, and blue dyes; and high caloric density. The taste is extremely bland without chemical intervention. These chemicals might make the food taste great, but they leave it nutritionally empty and health-destroying. Therefore, when a child consumes fast food, hunger actually increases. The craving pathway is set in motion to be a never-ending vicious cycle. You could term it the *vicious cookie cycle*.

Today, the average American, including children, consumes an estimated 115 pounds of sugar and sugar-laden processed foods each year. High sugar intake promotes oxidation and inflammation. This sets the tone for excess insulin production, which drives fat storage. Additionally, this level of poor food intake sets the stage for heart disease, cancer, and accelerated aging.

This is where most books on this subject would encourage you to eliminate certain foods and eat others. (And we'll get to that—don't worry!) But let's take it one step at a time. What we want you to focus on right now is the emotional connection you have with food.

The goal is to live your life in a healthy, four-part harmony. If we can recognize the root of unhealthy emotional attachments, we can make real lasting changes.

Your Spiritual Dimension

You probably have loved ones who have serious challenges physically, intellectually, or emotionally, yet *they have a good heart*. This is the way we describe the spiritual dimension of a person.

The spiritual dimension of life is the most important dimension, because it impacts the physical, emotional, and intellectual dimensions at all times. And we believe it's the part of you that can know God, or at least have a concept of who He is. But look—whatever you believe on this subject at this point is not our major concern. Our major concern is that your heart is open to receiving a new understanding of truth. This truth encompasses wellness in all these areas—physical, emotional, intellectual, and spiritual.

Stay with Us

Now that you've been reminded of what you knew deep inside— that you're a four-part being, designed to live in harmony—stay engaged with us on each dimension as we continue the journey.

For example, is your mind questioning or doubting something in this chapter? Dig deeper. Are your emotions freaking out, telling you change is not possible? Remind yourself that positive change is possible. Is your stomach growling or head hurting? Feed yourself something nutritious.

Most of all, don't shut us down. The journey to wellness might seem too hard—or even impossible. It's not. When thoughts, memories, fears, and feelings flare up, don't close your mind to the help we're going to offer.

If you're experiencing any of those "flare-ups" right now, that's wonderful! You're right where you need to be. When the flare-up occurs, issues are being *brought up* to be *brought out* of your life forever.

3

Living Between the Lines

Why do some people make remarkable improvements in their wellness and lifestyle, while others keep hitting a wall? Every success story we're familiar with, and we personally know hundreds, includes accountability. We're talking about a commitment to live between the lines.

But if the word *accountability* feels like a downer and deal-breaker, you've never experienced true, healthy accountability. Here are three questions to help you see and embrace this powerful ingredient of positive life change:

- What does it mean to be accountable?
- To whom are we to be accountable?
- How can we become consistently accountable?

What Does It Mean to Be Accountable?

To be accountable means to take responsibility for your actions, as well as your attitudes, beliefs, values, words, and actions.

When we're accountable, we're really creating an "accounting" for our "abilities."

Recognize that you have abilities that are uniquely your own. Your abilities are necessary for the world to have optimization and function. Without you doing your part (and fulfilling your abilities), the world (including your own personal world of family, friends, and colleagues) will not operate to its fullest.

To Whom Are We to Be Accountable?

Be very choosy about who you decide to be accountable to. First, we suggest, in addition to being accountable to our Creator, we should be accountable to ourselves. This means we face ourselves with total transparency and honesty—not in a denigrating or self-deprecating way, but in a way that causes us to admit to ourselves, *I am not the center of the universe.*

Many of our patients have a very one-sided accountability relationship with themselves—they only point out the negatives and failures, while ignoring the positives and successes.

Many health-related issues stem from a lack of self-love. Some people are basically committing suicide by diet choices and self-fulfilling spoken prophecies. And before you select other people as partners in your journey, make sure you assess your relationship with yourself.

Understanding that you have value is a prerequisite for this journey. If you have a negative view of yourself, you'll likely have a negative experience with accountability partners, even if they offer positive encouragement. (If you want to read our value pledge, go to www.SherwoodWellness.tv/bonus and receive this and other book bonuses.)

As human beings, we're designed to be in healthy relationships with other people. King Solomon said, "As iron sharpens iron, so a man sharpens the countenance of his friend" (Proverbs 27:17). Notice he used the word *friend.* Don't choose just anyone to speak into your life. Some words sharpen, and some words cut.

Choose friends wisely, as there are plenty of "false friends" around who'll suck the very life out of you. Now, we know you know what (and who) we are talking about. It's time to do some pruning for true growth. Choose someone who can hold you accountable at your weakest moments, someone you can lean on to stay the course with you against all odds. That's what it will take to continue to sharpen your iron and be the best *you* you can be.

We are to admonish others, with an attitude of love and compassion. And often this means speaking words that express conviction, challenge, and renewed affirmation. A true friend encourages excellence and continues to raise the bar of excellence. True friends lift you from mediocre to great on a daily basis.

If the idea of an accountability relationship sounds foreign or frightening, here's a good place to start. Look at your circle of friends and acquaintances and consider who you might encourage. Never offer challenge without first being invited, but encouragement is always welcome. There is a subtle principle here we don't want you to miss—give before you get. When you "give before you get," you'll never have to be concerned with getting because of the joy you receive from giving. This principle will serve you well in all areas of life.

How Can We Become Consistently Accountable?

Accountability means working with others to establish new habits. There's power in healthy, accountable relationships. We're social creatures, and we must be careful not to socialize with individuals who bring us down. We have all heard the phrase *misery loves company*. It's easy to fall into that trap, and growth stops when that trap is set.

The pursuit of wellness is a lot easier if you have others who believe as you believe and who are willing to discipline their lives in the same ways you are seeking to discipline your life.

We work out daily, usually early in the morning before we go to our offices. As part of our early-morning routine, we drink a high-protein shake that includes some fiber, greens, and various supplements. Not long ago, someone asked me about our early-morning smoothie. When I shared the ingredients, he said, "Remind me not to go to breakfast with you!" We both laughed. I could've misunderstood his remark, but I'd given a positive suggestion with good health benefits. He may choose to hear my message, weigh it against the outcomes in my life, and choose to act on it. But my responsibility was to tell the truth and provide insight. The other person's responsibility is to hear, consider, apply, and persevere in applying.

Remember, we're not here to convince you of anything. We're telling you about what has worked for others. It's your responsibility to receive and act on it.

Consider this as well: we love you enough to tell you the truth. But the truth is only accepted by those who are in pursuit of it. Not everyone wants to receive truth, because truth can create internal conflict. Recall what "truth" did to the person who asked about our morning routine. It created conflict.

Three Levels of Accountability

Several months ago, a man named Mitch came in to our clinic. He was a bit skeptical but wanted to address the issue of his weight. As a young man in his thirties with a young family, he had started thinking about his health.

His body fat percentage was around 25 percent, and we like to see numbers well below 20 percent. Mitch went through all our testing, including genetics and blood work, and in less than sixty days, his body fat percentage dropped by more than 7 percent.

How did he achieve such impressive results? He had three levels of accountability.

First, he made a choice to be accountable to his own convictions. Second, he decided to enlist us in pursuit of his goals, trusting us to give honest feedback, medical facts, and a plan to improve his overall wellness.

Third, his wife came on board. Although she was also skeptical, Mitch's decision sparked confidence in her. She joined him in the quest for total wellness as his accountability partner.

When it comes to accountability, there's no more powerful partner than your spouse.

Healthy Accountability with Your Spouse

In any relationship, change creates pressure—and pressure reveals weaknesses.

Obviously, your spouse has the potential to be a wonderful accountability partner. But conversations about change can also open up expressions of anger, frustration, and hurt, or worse—apathy.

So many people come to us seeking help. Most are desperate, and they've tried everything. One of the questions we ask them is, "Will your spouse be supportive?"

More often than not, we hear, "No, not really." That's heart-breaking, and we understand, because it breaks our hearts too. There's nothing we appreciate more than someone coming into the clinic with their spouse saying, "We're in this together."

It's always a win to have spouses work together. This action and bond has the ability to change total families and then spread into communities. The ultimate change would be a change in the health of our nation.

But even if you don't have support from your spouse, or if you're single, we want to assure you that success is possible. Even if everyone around you is eating cookies and chips, you can change your life and the lives of family and friends.

Sometimes, the greatest healer is the witness. When we witness a change in someone we want to see in ourselves, we'll grab hold of what we want. Being an example of a healthy lifestyle gives others the opportunity to see health—and seek it for themselves.

Find a trustworthy friend and share your dreams and goals. Ask that person to help you stick with your plan. Remember, first and foremost, your main accountability partner is you.

We've seen relationships strengthened through the process of accountability, even if at first the spouse wasn't on board. And if your spouse gave you this book to help you understand his or her hopes for a better life, please recognize the opportunity you have to better your relationship and improve your lives individually and together.

A woman came to us recently and began making healthy changes. Her husband supported her but didn't want to join her on the journey. He happened to be overweight and a type 2 diabetic. So we told her, "You need to do this for your husband."

"What do you mean?" she asked.

"Live this plan, consistently and quietly. Let him see health come into you, and we guarantee you he's gonna want what you have." She took our suggestion and began living as the witness.

Sure enough, several months later, he came to see us and declared, "I have to get some help." He was intrigued by her newfound zest for life, her level of energy, and her drive to get out of bed every day. She was no longer just showing up. She was shining.

Don't try to change anyone else; you can only change yourself. Let your actions speak. Actions, and results, are impossible to ignore.

What Is Healthy Accountability?

We love this definition of accountability: Accountability is not holding someone's feet to the fire and criticizing them. It's not a checklist you hold them to, and its not a focus on failures. Accountability is taking into *account* your *ability*. You have a special ability.

If I was on your accountability team, we'd first agree on the ability you possess. It's not my job to do something that's within your ability, but I can bring my questions, encouragement, and perspective.

I'd also remind you about certain truths.

None of us were designed to be overweight, sick, and relying on bottles of pills. Our bodies are struggling and crying out for help, because they were designed to stay healthy. So our ability, whether we believe it or not, is to seek wholeness and not settle for less.

When you took the "I Have Value Pledge," you held yourself to this higher standard. You, and your accountability partners, must be on the same page about your vision and beliefs.

A Healthy Alliance

Your accountability partner must want what's best for you and must believe you have the ability to achieve your full potential. He or she must be a friend and must not be afraid to be completely honest with you. You must demand this from anyone who really values the concept of genuine friendship. This realness must be communicated in love and with proper motives.

If you don't know your accountability partner, he or she is a mentor, not an accountability partner. There's a big difference. A mentor is someone you want to be like but don't really know. But an accountability partner is like a brother or sister.

Here's a good analogy: positive, life-changing accountability is like the members of a military unit who pledge allegiance to each other. They fight alongside each other, they defend each other, they protect each other, and they're willing to die for each other. That's true accountability.

If accountability conjures up an image of a drill sergeant who shouts, that's the wrong idea. A true ally helps you hold your "account" of love for yourself at a higher level.

This relationship doesn't have to take a lot of time in order to be effective. Simple text messages can work wonders to strengthen resolve and build encouragement.

We actually recommend "interviewing" people, like you would for a job. Share your goals, and share the philosophy you're learning in this book. (Give them a copy of this book.)

If they agree with this philosophy and want to be a part of your journey, then you can agree to begin. If they don't, that's okay. Not everyone has the time or energy to fill this role.

Ideally, you want to connect with someone who has a healthy lifestyle. This means if you and your spouse have both decided you need to change your lifestyle, you'll want to enlist someone, or another couple, who are further along the journey than you.

Our long-term vision, even with our clinic, is to create a community of accountability—a new normal that more and more people are encouraged to adopt. We need a new American lifestyle. And it starts with us.

Permission to Succeed

Many people think an accountability partner assumes the role of guardian and should check in with you about your goals. This view diminishes your ability. Instead, permission must come from you. First by giving yourself permission to succeed. And second by asking permission of your accountability partner.

"Do I have your permission to email (or text or call) you about my progress and challenges?"

The right person will not only agree, but they'll also reach out to you occasionally.

If you can't find an accountability partner right away, don't delay your pursuit.

- Go to our websites for blogs, videos, information, and articles—www.fmidr.com, www.wellnesslifeacademy.com, and www.sherwoodwellness.tv.
- If you're in the vicinity of our clinic, we offer a free monthly class for patients to stay engaged.
- A health club membership can be good for a basic level of accountability.

Remember, you don't need anyone else's permission to succeed. But you must give *yourself* permission, and all the help you are able to find.

A Skinny Fat Person

Cheryl was sick. And gaining weight.

She didn't know why and wondered if hormones were the cause. Cheryl came to see us with her husband, Travis, who happened to be an accomplished motorsports athlete.

When we asked Travis if he would like an evaluation, he answered, "I don't have any problems at all."

So, I (Dr. Michele) said to him, "You are probably a skinny fat person."

After the shock wore off, he replied, "I'm not either, I'm just fine."

I knew all too well by what he shared about his lifestyle—and by looking at him—that although he was slim, Travis wasn't healthy. He had a hidden yet evident spread around the middle and very thin extremities. A trained eye can spot sarcopenic obesity a mile away. *Sarcopenic obesity* is a term for "skinny fat."

We challenged him to have his blood work evaluated and to let us take a look at his biomarkers and the markers for systemic inflammation. Sure enough, he was almost a diabetic—a skinny, pancake-eating, athletic, diabetic. Internally, he was an absolute train wreck and didn't know it. Externally, he pulled off a physique that appeared athletic with a shirt that hid his midriff.

If a patient's blood work comes back showing diabetes, we are ethically obligated to prescribe the appropriate medication and treatment protocol to that person. *Appropriate* is the key word here. Most times, the appropriate medication is truth coupled with a good nutritional protocol. "Stop putting garbage in your mouth" may be a simpler way to put it.

With the rise of type 2 diabetes, caused by sugar, why aren't we calling this out more? We have to extinguish the cause and get sugar out of our lives. This diagnosis comes with a long laundry list of symptoms and an expensive pharmacy bill every month—not to mention increased insurance costs. The tragedy is that in most cases, type 2 diabetes is preventable.

Personally, we don't believe type 2 diabetes should exist when we really know how to stop it from happening in the first place. We have no idea why folks are focused on managing this condition when the mission should be eradication.

Watching and Listening

We turn patients around time after time after time, as long as they trust us and have accountability. And in a sense, you have to be your body's accountability partner. Listen to what your body is telling you, and pay attention to what your body is showing you.

Most of us sit down to food and inhale it. We don't chew it mindfully; we don't taste the flavors or note the textures. We often eat on the run in fifteen minutes or less. We fail to realize it takes twenty minutes for your brain to catch up with your stomach, so we're not even giving our bodies a chance to work right. That quick fifteen-minute window of indulgence has already put your system under stress. We must begin to slow down, chew our food, and listen to how food interacts when it lands in our stomachs and begins to undergo the processes of digestion.

It may seem odd to watch and listen to the action of food in our systems, but think of how your body responds to a hard workout. You're not sore the moment you finish your session, you're sore one or two days later. Food intake is much the same. The irritation and allergy can come days or weeks after eating the same irritant on a regular basis. Your stomach and intestinal track respond by becoming irritable, bloated, and/or full of gas. We have to pay attention.

Watch how your eyes may be bigger than your stomach. You pile your plate full and then follow the rules of the "clean your plate club." Your stomach is about the size of your fist. If you're not actively exercising and sitting down to large meals, you're falling prey to the vice of gluttony.

The *blood sugar blues* can be completely avoided. Take note of how you crave sugar about thirty to forty minutes after you just ate your last sugary food. Eating sugar creates a state of craving through imbalance with the hormone insulin. We call this the *vicious cookie cycle*.

When a system is in balance, it doesn't crave. The blood sugar blues are self-induced and can be overcome by listening to your body's response to the fuel you put in it.

Try limiting what you put on your plate to a few items at a time. One piece of protein (poultry, fish, eggs, or otherwise), one green, and one low-glycemic carbohydrate. You'll start to hear your body's voice as it handles the food and understand which one may cause issues. You'll come to know the answer to questions like: *Is it the dressing I piled on? The sugary treat I just ate? Is it emotion that's driving me to eat?*

Most of us go through life and don't pay any attention. We're like zombies much of the time, not really understanding why we do what we do. Can you relate?

We are accountable to our own physical bodies, intellect, emotions, and spirit.

The Power of Accountability

Travis and Cheryl made the decision to change and the decision to help each other achieve their wellness goals. Without each other's support, either of them could've easily gone off the rails.

In a few months, both turned their lives completely around. Their body fat dropped down into normal range with no medication.

His athleticism improved, and her energy improved—but best of all, their relationship improved. That's the power of healthy accountability.

Actions Speak Loudly

People watch what we do, not what we say.

If more physicians and medical professionals were living healthy lifestyles, more patients would come on board with them.

When you take action, you could impact your entire family, and even your neighborhood. Your actions will affect your children and your children's children. What are your actions communicating at this moment?

Children rarely do better than their parents. They rarely eat better than their parents. They look to their parents to lead. If you lead in a healthy direction, you can help make lasting change. After all, you're accountable for a share of their long-term habits, so make yours count.

A young couple came to our clinic to have their biomarkers and markers of inflammation checked. The wife had suffered years of a painful sickness, caused by a rare bacteria, and as a result was hooked on pain pills. All this contributed to significant weight gain through emotional eating and seeking comfort in food.

The doctors she saw wanted to give her more pills and told her she would have to live this way. She gave testimony to seeing seven different doctors who had all told her the same thing. She began to make our suggested lifestyle changes. We first had to get to the roots. She had to find out what was buried and make amends with it in order to continue on her journey to total wellness and freedom.

Her witness created curiosity in her husband. He questioned her about help for himself. She was the witness for long-lasting change. This witness infected first her husband and then the rest of her family.

She brought her husband in, he got on board, and they decided as a family to make some healthy changes. Their twelve-year-old son, Dillon, was also morbidly obese. He was following down the generation curse pathway of his mother. She realized how her own behavior was affecting the lives of her children and her spouse. As a family, they were able to get to the root before he turned thirteen years old. He could start his teens with a totality of wellness.

They all made tremendous progress. Probably the most rewarding part for us was to see their child, formally sedentary and addicted to video games, become active—riding his bike, running, and enjoying the outdoors.

The last time they went to their child's physical exam, the doctor said, "Who is this kid?" The transformation was, and still is, dramatic.

Don't Go Before Your Time

We don't particularly like funeral homes, but in one case, we made an exception. A couple who owns a funeral home happened to become our patients. Their turnaround was so dramatic that they have become champions of wellness in their community.

Their life message—even to potential funeral home customers—is, *We don't want you to die before your time. We want you to learn to live, so when you come to this place your family will celebrate a long life and many cherished memories.*

This couple had accountability partners with us and with each other. Now they're valued partners with others on their journey to wellness. They're creating a wellness community in their home town, spreading the wellness word, and they have shared their story in several local churches and community event centers.

Starting a Fire

Are you sick of being sick? Are you tired of medications?

Don't stop taking any prescriptions unless directed by a physician, but don't resign yourself to a future dependent on pills. Don't believe change is not possible! Change is the only thing you can truly count on. Change will happen, it's our part to shift it to a continual pattern of the positive variety.

Most importantly, don't go it alone. People are put into this world to specifically help you. Additionally, you were created uniquely to help someone else. That's the power of community and unity. When you have commonality in a purpose and passion, and you in turn join in unity with others, you have the powerful force of community.

Don't ask somebody else to change you. You make your decision. Once you decide, that's when you need people around you to keep that fire lit. It's like starting a fire—you have to keep throwing kindling on it, and then finally it will catch and begin to burn.

That's what an accountability partner does.

Imagine the impact your new choices will have on your life and the lives of others.

Time for PIES

We're not talking dessert here. It's time to start digging deeper to excavate your soon-to-be deep well of wellness.

As your own accountability partner, take a few minutes to talk with yourself about the four areas below. For each facet of your being, what do you want to change within, or about, each, and who might be healthy accountability partners?

- Physical: What do I want or need to change? Who would be able to help me?
- Intellectual: What do I need to learn? From where (or whom) is the best source of information?

- Emotional: Where do I need the most control or balance? Who have I seen exhibit the qualities I want?
- Spiritual: What do I need most in this dimension? Who is in the best person to speak with?

4

Frauds Hinder Wellness

WE'RE WILLING TO BET YOU'VE TRIED TO LOSE WEIGHT OR improve some aspect of your health before. Most people in the Western world have tried many fad diets, quick fixes, and even weight loss/diet pills. Most have failed and ended up right back where they started or even worse off.

What's responsible for this failure? What hinders the path to health and healing when the road is clear? We know what to do, and we often know how to do it, but we can't seem to stay the course.

What prevents us from being truly whole in spirit, mind, emotions, and body? What are the roadblocks that hinder our progress toward wellness? What are the strong holds that derail us and pull us off course and ruin our best efforts?

Perhaps it's a new kind of fraud. Fraud with an *S*. A *frauds* that sneaks into our lives like a serpent in the night, coming to kill, steal and destroy our well-being.

FRAUDS is an acronym for:

F = Fear
R = Resentment
A = Anger

U = Unforgiveness

D = Disappointment

S = Shame

We're talking about deep-seated patterns and struggles, not temporary displays of emotion linked to a particular circumstance. These patterns and struggles are often set in motion in the mind of the young and cripple the well-being of the adult. The conscious mind knows the solution, yet the deep-seated patterns rule the behaviors and daily choices the "infected" individual makes.

An infection can be a simple statement. For example, the statement "You're ugly" places a string of worthlessness and destructive patterning in the nervous system of the receiver of those words. This wound seeks comfort, most often in food but also sometimes in drugs, alcohol, sex addiction, and the list goes on.

The receiver is infected with a negative voice that repeats day after day, "You're ugly." If the root issue isn't addressed with truth and love, comfort-seeking and self-medicating behavior comes to life. Of course, the person does not set out to intentionally destroy oneself. He or she is simply looking for pain relief and the feeling of self-acceptance the mind is unable to provide.

The statement "You may forget what someone said, but you never forget how they made you feel" is true. Emotions can root themselves in the barracks of your mind and hack your health through negative behavior and life-destroying choices. We call these the "spiritual roots" of sickness and disease.

Let's Dig Up Some Roots

How do roots show up? What do they look like?

We all know people who seem to be perpetually fearful. They may not identify the feeling as a fear but will admit to being a "worrier" or continually expecting something bad to happen. The chronic worrier usually points to the world with the idea, "See, there's plenty to be worried about!"

The ability to shift gears from worry to joy is an impossibility. This person will deny depression but definitely doesn't live within happiness. He or she seeks comfort, most often in food and second, third, and otherwise in drugs, alcohol, sex addiction, and the list goes on. Our main focus in this book is the behavior of gluttony and addiction to comfort food.

Everyone knows someone who's a powder keg of anger just waiting to explode. They may justify their anger by saying they "get over it" quickly, but others know better. They often become abusers, even justifying their abuse. And they're always hurting themselves.

They hurt themselves in a multitude of ways: destroying relationships and then feeling the shame and guilt. They place blame on themselves in negative and destructive ways, spiraling into behaviors of comfort, most often in food, and second, third, and otherwise in drugs, alcohol, sex addiction, and the list goes on. Are you starting to see a repetitive pattern? Can you see how these fickle emotions called *spiritual roots* wreak havoc on the very health we pray for? They set root and give sprouts to shoots of other negative emotions.

We pray for deliverance yet never get rid of the root. The behavior continues to destroy us. We are destroying ourselves down to the very core of our DNA. Yes that's right. We can influence our genes by how we behave.

We all know people who can't seem to let go of a hurt, even if it happened three or four decades ago, or even in the first five years of age. They continue to want vengeance on the person who did them wrong or live in a loathing state of the "what dad did" syndrome—my parents abandoned me, my brother abused me, and the list goes on. These people are usually very difficult to love and insulate themselves against genuine compassion.

In their heart of hearts, it's really what they want in the first place—love.

You probably know someone who deeply resents what they consider to be an injustice, which left them lacking, impoverished, denied, or "pulled down a rung" on the social or economic ladder. They chalk all their personal failures up to something done *to* them. Rarely do these people have any moments of exhilarating hope, and they usually live in a chronic state of holding on to the past as if it's the present. The person who was part of the root may have long since passed away and, in many cases, may not even live in the same city. We all know it's as hard to undo a rumor as it is to unring a bell. We can identify with falsehoods and never get past them. The spiritual stronghold gets hold of us on the inside and changes behavior, often spiraling them into behaviors of comfort, most often in food, and second, third, and otherwise: drugs, alcohol, sex addiction and the list goes on.

Everyone knows people who can seldom be pleased—by anyone or about anything. They may manifest this by being constantly critical, cynical, frustrated, or fault-finding. They live in a state of abiding gloom without much joy. They have an antagonistic attitude no matter what the circumstance. They can find conflict in any conversation and go down a repetitive path that spirals into a toxic cesspool of ridiculousness, affecting whomever they're in relationship with in a negative way. Often, they end up spiraling into behaviors of comfort, most often in food, and second, third, and otherwise in drugs, alcohol, sex addiction, and the list goes on.

Yes, the attributes of FRAUDS are longstanding traits in some people and even in communities of people and families. They can be generational. How many times have you heard, "I don't want to be like my mother was?" or "I sure don't want to be like Dad?" As time goes on, where do we end up if we don't stay awake and conscious of what's driving our behavior and actions?

In each example above, our question to you is: *Are you one of those people?*

Fraudulent thinking leads a person to believe lies: *no person can ever experience perfect health; people need pills to produce health; there is no other way.* Those who buy into lies often have roots of fraudulent behavior in their heart, and they don't even know of their serious infection.

Frauds pulls people away from the truth.

We're going to unravel the frauds and uncover why food has become the false comforter. Our goal is for you to experience freedom from emotional, spiritual, and physical sickness and disease. After all, that's our goal, right? We want healthy, joy-filled, passionate days without unnecessary suffering.

Generational Frauds

Let's look at generational curses. We spoke briefly about not wanting to be like Mom or Dad. Remember, we're not pointing fingers at anyone. We're unroofing what we experience as blockages to healing in our patients and in people who are seeking total healing. Many patients who come to us for care and healing appear to have roots of frauds that are *generational.* This means that the person was taught, directly or inadvertently, to *be* fearful, resentful, angry, unforgiving, or continually disappointed because a parent, grandparent, or other family figure routinely displayed similar responses to life.

A child is a sponge for learning, and this learning is mostly from example. Most of the skills we develop in life we learn by copying the behavior of others.

Have you ever stopped for a moment to ask, "Why do I do what I do?"—down to the very act of brushing your teeth, getting dressed, or driving a car? Most of us haven't examined the root causes and influences, especially when it comes to how we respond and act in this event we call *life*. Our patterns of behavior just "do" us.

Stop and think about it. If Dad struck Mom in abusive anger because he saw Grandpa strike Grandma in abusive anger, what's the likelihood the child will grow up thinking it's acceptable to strike a spouse if anger is felt?

If Mom is a constant worrier, could it be she learned that behavior from her mother? What will be the child's tendency growing up?

If Dad and Mom are overweight, it may be attributed by them, and other members in the family, to "being of stocky-built people" who just happened to like lots of pasta and breads loaded with butter and creamy sauces.

What's likely on their dinner table? What's a child in their home likely to grow up eating and craving as "comfort food" as an adult?

Patients come into our clinic every week seeking weight loss and ask us, "Why are you talking about mindset and emotions? I just want to lose some weight."

The answer is quite clear. Most know "what to do" but don't do it. If they do it, they do it for a limited time. The path to health is straight and narrow, and very few find it. If there's a root of pain and dysfunction, how long can a person stay the course? How long until the ingrained infectious behavior rooted somewhere in frauds shows back up?

That's why we have two big reasons for talking about emotions and mindset.

First, because you want to enjoy health in four-part harmony. What good is physical health without emotional health? What good is intellectual mastery without spiritual peace? We are interconnected beings. One part is not healthy and completely whole without the sum of all of its parts.

Second, the difference between success and failure is dealing with all four facets of our design. That's right. We must deal with all four facets of our being. If we neglect even a fraction of one, we won't reach our max potential of well-being.

Let's take a look at each of the six aspects of FRAUDS.

Fear

Fear keeps you out of trouble. Before you pull out from a traffic light, you look left and right, based on a healthy fear of harm. But fear can keep you *in* trouble. It can paralyze you.

We all understand the feeling of fear. But we don't often understand its roots or how to be free from it.

Fear is driven in the media today. There's fear of terrorism, fear of an economic crash, fear of bad news, and fear of illness. Many of our patients have a fear of being fat. I (Michele) experienced this, with the intense fear of being fat driving my emotional engine.

My adopted father was morbidly obese. He hated himself. He was miserable in mind and spirit. I became rigid in my mindset around food, afraid of eating and especially fearful of eating any sort of fat. I maintained a ridiculously low body weight, counting calories and eliminating fat from anything I ate. Many days, I would survive on a can of green beans and tomatoes.

I was a tremendous athlete and addicted to exercise, partly motivated by my fears. Exercise was my escape from dealing with negative emotions and was the way I found control over my fear of obesity.

When I (Mark) was growing up, I struggled with approval. I still do, to some extent. The fear of rejection goes back to childhood—being an only child, adopted, and not one of the cool guys in school.

If you know there is something you need to do, you know there will be fear. You have to do it even if you are afraid. Growth happens when you step outside of your comfort zone. You can't grow standing still.

If fear stops you, it wins. Fear is a normal part of living. Experiencing fear means you're human. So the good news is, if you feel fear about your journey to wellness, welcome to the club! We've been there.

To acknowledge fear is one thing; to give it power is another. It's much like the stress response coined by Dr. Hanse Selye when he coined the term General Adaptation Syndrome (GAS). In his teaching, he clearly outlined how the stress response can become chronic and "normal." When it becomes "normal" to be stressed out, we simply forget how to relax, and then we run out of "GAS." Obviously, we have greatly simplified this research, but you get the idea. Living with chronic stress will destroy your health. The same is true with chronic fear.

Acknowledge that that fear is normal and temporary. If you take steps forward, you can control your fear. If you don't get it under control, it will control you.

Resentment

Have you ever had the experience of seeing someone you know and wanting to walk the other way? That's resentment. When you hear the name of someone who hurt you and want to cause them the pain they caused you, that's resentment. When you read about someone's success in the newspaper and feel bad about your failure to accomplish your goals, that's self-resentment.

We can carry resentment and not even know it's there. It gets rooted deep and festers like a pimple.

I (Michele) look back on the hurts I experienced in my younger years. I suffered wounds of abandonment, abusive relationships, personal injury, and homelessness. I never understood my father's health conditions. Internal resentment of misunderstanding led to intense anger. Little did I realize resentment is like an infection that won't heal. Eventually the wound of resentment turns into anger. The pus of resentment breeds the next toxic emotion that affects behavior.

Anger

It's okay to have the emotion of anger. Some define anger as the feeling that something is wrong and needs to be made right.

Anger is real and shouldn't be dismissed or repressed. Think of the good that's come from people acting out of righteous anger: defending the defenseless, bringing justice, and standing against evil.

You can be angry at another person, and that's normal, but don't let the anger become chronic. Anger will drive our blood pressure up, which can drive up our cortisol, and our stress hormones will increase chronically. Cortisol drives blood sugar, and when blood sugar goes up, it drives insulin, and when insulin is up in a chronic way, there are two responses: you begin to store fat, and you become inflamed. Anger is a powerful emotion that, left unchecked, will lend to a path of destruction—destruction of self and of others.

In our view, chronic anger is a disease . . . and a precursor to disease.

For some, a shield of fat becomes their coat of armor—an attempt to form a protective shield from emotional un-wellness or the inability to face the root of our pain.

Here's an example to ponder. In the early spring of last year, a young man came to see us for help with his weight. As he told us, he had tried every diet and weight-loss strategy and even tried a few types of diet pills. He was the typical person who may lose a few pounds and gain it back, plus a few. He turned to us as his last hope.

In order to get to the root, we like to ask a lot of questions. Once you understand an individual's history, the problem reveals itself. We strive to know our patients and the challenges they face. After all, we want success.

He was allowed the platform without interruption, and we were given the chance to hear his full story for the first time. At the conclusion, we asked a few questions about the reason he came: weight loss.

We asked, "How long have you struggled with weight?"

"Since childhood."

"Did your parents show any favoritism toward you or your sibling?"

"Yes, my brother was their favorite."

"Did he struggle with weight?"

"No." We could see emotions rising up.

Bingo. We were onto something. So we asked, "How did your parents handle that with you?"

"Well, my parents used to encourage me to lose weight . . . and be more like my brother."

We could feel the weight of those words and the burden he had carried, even though his parents had long since passed. He went on to marry a woman who seemed to be able to eat anything she wanted and not gain weight. She wasn't healthy by any means, but she was slim. She was on five different medications and had a multitude of health issues, but she didn't carry the lack of self-esteem he did from being overweight.

When she told him he needed to lose weight, all the fear, resentment, and anger came rushing back like a bad dream. The bad dream was his childhood memory of being shamed for being overweight. This was the root of his stronghold. This was the root of his food addiction. This behavior continued to drive him back to the place he didn't want to be. In fact, every time he would try to lose weight, he always rebounded with a few extra pounds. He had never faced where the issues came from.

No harm was intended, but because of the baggage he carried, his wife's words were misinterpreted. We had to dive in and get to the root.

Sometimes we have to go back to our childhood years, our teenage years, or to the first time we were hurt. Deeply hurt. "Who hurt you the worst?" we often ask. Many times we discover the root of our problem is from childhood, our first "best friend," or our first "true love."

Let's Take a Break

Whether you're reading this book for your own journey to wellness or as an accountability partner, let's pause and process what we've covered in this chapter so far.

There may be painful emotional explosions going off inside you as you read this. If so, please know this is normal and healthy. It's time for introspection and placing the magnifying glass on deep-seated wounds.

Identifying the root cause is part of the process and part of the progress. You may experience fear, resentment, anger, unforgiveness, and echoes of disappointment like you haven't in years.

When these feelings come up, are you tempted to medicate those feelings with food? Are you seeking comfort in all the wrong places? It's easy to live in denial and on the run. It's easy to grab a quick fix and stuff feelings. It's easy to avoid the internal warfare. At least it seems easy, until all *health* breaks loose. When health breaks loose and becomes laden with sickness and disease, that's what gets our attention.

Obesity kills, it hurts, and it's emotionally devastating. It will eventually get our attention. The roots eventually have to be dealt with. They have to be dealt with in order to be completely and totally well.

If you found yourself saying yes to food as a medication or a comfort, there's a time of detox ahead—withdrawal from the drug of food. There's an answer, and there's a way out.

Cupcakes and cocaine—neither want to let go of you. So take a breath. Give yourself a break. Trust us. You're on a proven path to wellness.

Maybe you feel conflicted because you want to change your life, but you know change will be difficult. Stay with us. Don't sabotage your own desires.

As we say, living a lifestyle of health and wellness is hard, but being overweight and being sick is harder.

You must choose your "hard." The path to health and wellness is narrow; very few find it. The ones who do are totally free—free from food addictions that drive the cycles of unhealthy behaviors leading to obesity, chronic sickness, and disease.

Emotions often become ugliest right before a breakthrough. FRAUDS unveil themselves with a vengeance, often more strongly than ever before, because this time, they're not being quieted with food.

FRAUDS are designed to steal your life away, and they don't want to let go. They must be faced head-on and dealt with. Once we have healthy tools in place, emotions no longer have a hold on our lives. Our choices change as our behaviors change, and the roots that once gave emotions life are now extinguished.

Remember, emotions talk—and might even scream—at you, but they will never hurt you unless you let them. Keep walking forward. Emotions often surface like layers of an onion until the last layer has been swept away. It takes time, patience, and most of all self-love.

For Accountability Partners

If you're reading this as an accountability partner, consider the role of fear, resentment, anger, unforgiveness, and shame in your own life—especially when it comes to the unhealthy habits you can't seem to break and the resolutions you can't seem to keep.

Then put yourself in the shoes of the person you're partnering with.

In my own life, I (Michele) had to resolve my childhood issues before I could really help someone else authentically. Of course, I could give logical advice, but until I had uprooted the toxic roots that kept me reeling in some negative behaviors, I knew I couldn't completely help someone else.

Through my journey, I faced the fear of abandonment, the resentment of betrayal and abuse by my early relationships, and the anger I had pent up inside from failures and rejections. I had so much unforgiveness inside from all of the wounds I was carrying, I isolated myself from the human race because no one was safe.

I realized one day that my life was one big disappointment and I was completely and utterly ashamed of it all.

The only thing I could bear witness to was the bitterness and pain I felt at the end of every day. That's no way to help others. I had to seek and find healing for myself first—one day at a time.

I walked through the valleys of what I thought was the shadow of death. I learned not to fear; I learned to forgive. I had to forgive myself first in order to forgive others. The journey was long, tears were shed, toxic emotions were unroofed, and the power I used to give them was now dead.

The journey at the end of the rainbow led to ultimate freedom. Had I not chosen to be accountable to myself first, I couldn't truly know what another person was going through—nor could I understand the path of true freedom and healing for them.

Remember, this is a lifestyle change. There will be a period of adjustment: physically, intellectually, emotionally, and spiritually.

Unforgiveness

Why not begin with you? Are you willing to forgive yourself?

You can't give what you don't have.

We don't expect you to be perfect. We sure aren't. But what we expect, and what you should expect, is perfect effort. This means when you fall down, there are three choices. Number one, you can lie there while everyone else moves on and let resentment turn to anger. Number two, you can cry. And cry.

And stay in the sadness and wallow in the pain. But there's a third option.

You can dust yourself off and say, "Well, I fell. It happens sometimes when you move. It can easily happen when you change directions. And I'm human. So I choose to forgive myself and get up."

We've all made mistakes. But not everyone forgives themselves.

Have you put a limit on the number of times you forgive others? Maybe that's because you've put a limit on forgiving yourself. Sometimes it's much more difficult to forgive yourself than it is to forgive someone else.

That's why we start with this question: will you forgive yourself? Are you willing to at least say the words out loud?

"I forgive myself."

Even a whisper is a beginning. Now you may choose to also say, "God, please forgive me, and help me forgive those who hurt me."

Congratulations. You're beginning. You're moving through the layers of fraud.

Disappointment

The long-term effects of fear, resentment, anger, and unfor-giveness are an outlook of continual disappointment. Sounds pretty terrible. But billions of people experience this state of mind.

Unforgiveness leads into disappointment. Disappointment leads to despair. We can watch someone come into our office and know they're in despair by the way they carry themselves. Shoulders are slumped, eyes don't engage.

It almost makes us understand why a caring physician would want to prescribe some antidepressant pills for someone in this state. But we know these medications will only lead to weight gain and delay the person from addressing the deeper issues holding them back. Often, these medications lead to a sense of being numb and shielded from emotional pain. They don't provide active tools in the toolbox to deal with the roots of the problem.

We prescribe a unique tool to every one of our patients: *healing words*.

We all know that words can heal or kill. Replacing your toxic vocabulary will instantly start an internal healing process.

We recommend replacements for words like these: "I'm a victim of my father's alcoholism," "I'm fat and I'm ugly," "I'm a product of my father's destructive past."

Words create. King Solomon said, "Death and life are in the power of the tongue" (Proverbs 18:21). If we asked you to think of a big steak and baked potato, you'd picture it in your mind because words create. The pictures we create with our words stick with us and can shape our future.

For example, we'll say to a patient, "The sun's out today!" The patient might answer, "Yeah but it's a little cold."

Or: "That's a beautiful color on you." "Yes, but I didn't get my hair done today."

Sound familiar? In a ten-minute conversation, you can learn a lot about someone and their level of disappointment. Conversations also reveal our deepest disappointments with ourselves.

Shame

Disappointment and despair lead to the shame. All the areas we highlighted above ultimately relate to how we respond to the ups and downs of life. We are ashamed of our actions and even ashamed of life's twists and turns. And that's all we ever see in the mirror. Instead of seeing a person who's overcoming, we see a person who's overcome.

Humor is one way people hide shame. People who hide shame often over-talk and make fun of themselves. They're always hiding, which is easy to do on social media. The problem is, social media is a breeding ground for comparison and shame.

If someone is living in chronic shame, of course you know they're disappointed, they're angry at someone, and they haven't forgiven themselves.

All together, FRAUDS lie—about who you truly are.

Freedom from FRAUDS

I (Michele) had to walk through the stages of FRAUDS myself to evaluate why I did what I did and where my emotional drive came from. I was surviving and not truly living. In fact, I was dying inside.

Growing up, we lived in a house in the country where all the neighbors had really nice houses. Except us. My family was very poor. Our yard was unmowed and unkempt. I was ashamed of being poor.

I carried this shame through life. My father was very overweight, and both my parents were older, which also embarrassed me. But I kept it inside and kept busy taking care of them. At some point in life you have to look back and ask, "Where are all these toxic emotions coming from?"

My story is probably best described as *fifty years bitter, now fifty times better.*

All the good food in the world may not make you healthy if you're emotionally sick or intoxicating yourself with FRAUDS.

It's not only what we eat but what's eating us.

Going Back in Time

Why does a person look to food for comfort? Because they learned the habit as a child or soon thereafter. For many, food was one of the few sources of happiness.

Let's go back even further.

Have you ever thought about the significant role food has played in our history? Whether you believe the Bible story or not, we can agree it's quite interesting that in the garden of Eden, humankind traded paradise for a bite of food.

A momentary pleasure on the taste buds led to a much shorter and more painful life. Or, as we say today, *a moment on the lips, a lifetime on the hips*. But this, too, is a lie. Adam and Eve experienced *fear*. More specifically, fear of missing out. They had plenty of delicious food to eat, yet they chose to disobey. They believed the lie that if they didn't eat the forbidden fruit, their lives would somehow fall short.

They *resented* God and then each other, and they would go on to resent themselves. *Anger* followed, along with *unforgiveness*. That one decision about food brought immense despair. And if you continue reading the story, you'll see how their decision wreaked havoc on their children, and generations to come. The very first murder in recorded history involved food.

Suddenly they felt a strange, horrible sensation. *Shame*. Prior to their sneaky snack, they only experienced unconditional love. Now they were ashamed of themselves.

The issue isn't food, although it remains a temptation. The issue is the ability to love yourself, which empowers you to love others.

We sometimes use the analogy of cocaine to describe the challenge of overcoming the addiction to food as comfort. If you're addicted to cocaine, you can quit and never invest in it again. You can walk away from the group of people you associated with to partake in the habit. Once the door is closed, you are less likely to go back.

When it comes to breaking free from the emotions tied to food and food addiction, these are much harder to break, since you have to eat every day. And if you're addicted to food, you can't stop eating. You must change how and *why* you eat. The roots of behavior around food have to be pulled out and fully analyzed in order for you to be set completely free.

Cheat Days

When it comes to lifestyle, we don't diet. We choose to live a healthy life every day. We are often asked the question, "What do you eat on your cheat days?" Let's just settle the question right here.

Cheating is never okay. Not in your marriage, not in your finances, not on your taxes, and not in anything else in your life. So why do we believe there's no harm in cheating on our nutrition?

In the body-building world, a cheat day was a day to eat whatever you wanted for twenty-four hours and then get back on your plan. As we got smarter in athletics, we realized that cheat days weren't really a good thing. The negative consequences with cheat days were delayed healing time, fatigue, changes in weight, increased body fat, stomach and bowel upset, and more.

But if you splurged on foods that were healthier, you could get off your plan and get back on with fewer negative consequences.

Most people don't "cheat" with healthy food, they binge with gluttonous behaviors for a day and call it a "cheat day." But cheating is never okay and never good for you. How can something bad be good for you?

You might be wondering, *Gosh, are you guys the food police?*

Absolutely not. But in this book, we hope to be the FRAUDS police. Patterns of cheating yourself out of healthy eating (and a healthy life) can actually kick start the whole cycle of fear, resentment, anger, unforgiveness, disappointment, and shame. We hope to educate you to this fact so you can protect yourself.

Our only motivation is to spare you the pain from unhealthy behaviors and choices and see your life improve.

One cheat day becomes two, which often becomes a week, a month, a year, and then a lifetime. This journey is not a Daniel Fast or a New Year's resolution. We want you to feel better every single day.

Do you drive your car like you eat? In other words, do you stay in your lane *most* of the time, or *all* of the time? We don't tempt fate with our driving habits, so why would we do it with our health? You wouldn't put sugar in the gas tank of your car, would you? If the answer was yes, you'd find it wouldn't get you very far down the road. If the answer was no, then why would you put it in your own metabolic engine?

If all of the world put sugar in their gas tanks, we would no doubt improve our cardiovascular health, as everyone would soon be forced to walk or ride bikes.

My New Normal

It's normal to have fear, resentment, anger, unforgiveness, disappointment, and shame. But this doesn't have to be *your* normal.

Imagine being free from toxic emotions and free from toxic foods. Imagine your new normal of health and peace.

FRAUDS can steal your true identity.

You were designed to be well—physically, intellectually, emotionally, and spiritually. That's who you really are. You're not a fat person, a weak person, or a failure. The real you is seeking health. Your body heals itself relentlessly day after day. By design, it's designed to heal. Let's stop standing in its way.

In future chapters, we're going to address specific areas of physical health. But we encourage you to reread this chapter, write notes, meditate, and pray prayers as long as is needed to build up your true identity and recognize FRAUDS.

What you're seeking won't just come from food. Ultimately, we were designed for freedom and vitality.

Facing FRAUDS

As in the previous chapter, we want you to ponder and contemplate some thoughts. Take some time to look for FRAUDS in your life, and write down how each of these might be affecting your physical, intellectual, emotional, and spiritual health. To reach your destination, you need to identify unhealthy baggage, and pull it out by the root.

- Fear: What are my greatest fears?
- Resentment: Do I resent anyone? When I hear the name _____, I get really upset.
- Anger: What really angers me? Is it someone?
- Unforgiveness: Who do I need to forgive?
- Disappointment: Does disappointment rule my outlook on life?
- Shame: Am I living in shame? Am I ashamed of the way I look, the way I feel, the relationships I have chosen, or my career path?

Take your time answering the questions above. This is the beginning stage of your breakthrough to optimum wellness.

DISEASES WE DREAD AND WHAT TO DO INSTEAD

The only antidote for fear, and for all the FRAUDS we have discussed thus far, is truth.

Congratulations on pressing through fear and venturing into reading about diseases we dread. In this chapter, we're going to bring truth to light, with the goal of removing irrational fears and unnecessary dread.

Remember, your body was designed to be healthy and stay that way. With proper care and feeding, your health can improve. Think about all of the times you've watched wounds heal with only a remnant of a scar as witness to a past event.

Why Aren't We Healthier?
In the Western world, we have an unbelievable array of good food to eat, pure water to drink, sufficient energy sources, access to sound information, reliable communication systems, and trained medical personnel. The list could go on and on.

In addition, we have all sorts of programs to lose weight, build strength, and reduce stress. We have fitness centers, weight-loss centers, and trainers of all types. If you live in a rural community, you can access many of these programs online. Even so, Americans are more obese than ever. Metabolic syndrome is on the rise.

Metabolic syndrome is the precursor to type 2 diabetes and carries at least three of its five risk factors: high blood sugar, central obesity (fat around the middle of even a "skinny" person can spell trouble), high triglycerides, high blood pressure, and low HDL (high density lipoproteins).

These risk factors are common in our society today and are medicated as individual disease states, when they should be totaled up for a clear picture of how severely inflamed and sick the individual is.

Obesity is a contributing factor to many diseases and chronic ailments. Serious diseases—heart disease, cancer, diabetes—are still very prevalent, and in some cases they are escalating in numbers and severity. While we've made many strides in new medical protocols, procedures, and medicines, we as Americans are consuming an *increasing* amount of antacids and digestive aids, pain killers, mood elevators (uppers and downers), and sleeping pills.

Tragically, many of these diseases and ailments are completely preventable. So why are we so ill when we have so many resources? In addition to the FRAUDS described in the previous chapter, there are three main reasons:

Reason #1: A Lack of Good Information

Although more information is available to us than ever before, most people don't know where to find the information they really need and aren't sure they'll understand it when they read it. Further, most people aren't sure they can trust the source of the information, so they don't take action.

Information is only good if a person can understand it and see a way to apply it.

There is also a high percentage of people who adopt the policy of "no news is good news." Unless a person is in a great deal of discomfort, most won't seek help. Most think, *this will pass, I'm just getting old,* or *There's probably not anything a doctor can help me with anyway.* This applies to all forms of care—including emotional, psychological, and spiritual.

We must remind you of what you already know: ignorance is not bliss.

Many are woefully inept in their desire to prevent ailments or to address ailments while they're still in minor and curable states.

We're also easily persuaded thinking foods or activities we enjoy can't possibly be bad for us, rather than believing the facts based on good information.

Reason #2: A Lack of Vision

We're not talking about eyesight. We're talking about having a hope for the future and an understanding of our human potential.

Do you have a mental picture of what you might feel like if you truly attained wellness? Do you have an inner vision of what your life would be like if you were totally free from the fraud factors identified in the previous chapter?

Reason #3: Lack of a Plan

Many people need help developing a workable plan to get from Point A (where they are) to Point B (where they truly want to be).

When we began our clinic, we believed we would be dealing with people primarily at the "let's make a workable plan" level. Instead, we found the majority of our time was spent, at least in our first few meetings with a new patient, at the level of providing good information and presenting a "vision" of wellness.

So we now ask during our first appointments:

- What do you know about health and wellness?
- Do you have a vision for just how "well" you might be, in all areas of your life (physical, intellectual, emotional, and spiritual), with each area integrated at maximum levels of health?
- Do you want to make a plan to move from where you are to where you want to be?

How well can you answer the above questions?

In the following chapters, we're going to present the truth about eight of the diseases we dread the most. Instead of avoidance and fear, we're going to offer straight talk and hope.

You're ready for straight talk and hope.

5

Cardiovascular Disease

CARDIOVASCULAR DISEASE IS OFTEN KNOWN AS CORONARY artery disease (CAD), a fancy name for heart disease or hardening of the arteries.

If the circulatory highway system (arterial) in your body isn't treated right, with the right nutrition and proper lifestyle, these highways become inflamed, stiff, and hard, and they fill up with plaque. Artery walls become thin and cracked and eventually become unstable, leading to heart attack or stroke (heart attack of the brain). We all know life is carried in the blood, in the form of nutrients and oxygen. If the arteries can no longer move these important components to the peripheral tissues, cells start to die.

How can stiff, inflamed, cracked, and unstable arteries meet the high nutrient demand our bodies are under every day? When arteries are subject to years of ongoing stress from the standard American diet, plaque forms in their walls. This plaque is a byproduct of cholesterol that gets under the endothelial lining and becomes oxidized by the immune system. The immune system launches a protective response, calling in its troops to prepare for further attack. These immune cells try to destroy the invasion of cholesterol by releasing a product similar to bleach. That's right—when they try to bleach the incoming invaders, the invaders become oxidized, and the immune cells eat the invaders and grow into large cells called foam cells. These foam cells are the beginning stages of plaque formation.

Plaque formation starts with growing, inflamed foam cells. The arteries widen first in their attempt to keep the vessel lumen open. When the artery can no longer expand outward, it becomes stiff and resistant. The vessel then starts to narrow the lumen, because the plaque has nowhere else to go. If you've had a heart attack, you most likely have plaque. In fact, you have unstable plaque. That plaque isn't just in the arteries of your heart, it's in the arteries of your whole system.

The majority of cardiovascular disease deaths are related to coronary artery disease. There are other causes of death related to cardiovascular disease or HOCM—hypertrophic cardio-myopathy, dilated cardiomyopathies, and atrial/ventricular dysrhythmias.

Statistically, cardiovascular disease has been the number one killer of men and women for several years. However, as recently as the year 1900, cardiovascular disease wasn't the number one killer; it was around eight or nine. This change is indicative of people's nutritional habits.

In the year 1900, Americans consumed as much as 50 percent fat in their diets. This makes sense, because most people ate natural, fresh foods from their farms as well as meats they raised or hunted. Genetically modified organisms (GMOs) didn't exist. People simply ate what God made. They ate what grew from the ground and on trees, walked on land, or swam in the ocean. This food was full of nutrients, enzymes, and the appropriate ratios for the balance of protein, carbohydrates, and fats. Fake fats, trans fats, or hydrogenated oils didn't exist. Food was found in its natural form. Food was truly organic, with no pesticides, hormones, antibiotics, preservatives, gluten, MSG, fillers, or dyes.

Sure, generally speaking, most people didn't live as long. But this was mainly due to the presence of infectious diseases and viruses and relatively crude health care. And one hundred years later, cardiovascular disease is the number one killer, with cancer in second place.

We went from diets consisting of up to 50 percent fat to less than 20 percent fat. Interestingly, the "fat-free" food craze of recent decades, with the introduction of countless pills for every complaint, seems to have made our hearts less healthy.

Are we living longer per capita by age? Yes, technically our bodies are surviving more years, on average. But are we "living" longer? The answer is no. Life is really meant to be *lived* instead of *died.* Think about that statement for a moment. Are you *living* through life or *dying* through life?

Here's some good news. Cardiovascular disease can be prevented, slowed to a screeching halt, or reversed, almost 100 percent of the time with proper nutrition, testing, and awareness. We don't have to have plaque build-up in our arteries; it's not a birthright.

Cholesterol doesn't tell the whole story. More than half of cardiovascular events occur in people with normal cholesterol.

Most cardiovascular events occur with blockages in arteries that are half blockages, not full. But we usually don't see the blockages until they become full.

Maybe we've been asking the wrong question, which means we've gotten the wrong answer. Instead of asking how we treat heart disease, we should be asking, *how can we prevent it?*

Resigned or Resolute?

When people are resigned to the idea of eventually living with cardiovascular disease, they often do. Are there some mystical powers at work? No. But when people believe they have no choice in the matter, they won't make other choices toward prevention. Many live with an attitude of *it is what it is, or it just is.*

A hopeful, preventive approach to cardiovascular disease reduces fear. At least 80 percent of the risk factors for cardiovascular disease are managed by what we do. If I prescribed you a pill to reduce your chance of a heart attack by 80 percent, would you take it?

As part of our diagnostics, we utilize the Cleveland HeartLab inflammatory risk factor evaluation. The markers in this test provide an inside view of what's happening to your vascular system through a blood test. The markers are as follows:

- Myeloperoxidase (MPO) is a vascular-specific inflammatory enzyme released by white blood cells into the bloodstream in response to vulnerable plaque, erosions, or fissures in the artery wall. Elevated levels of MPO are associated with risk of cardiac events and may assist in cardiovascular risk prediction.
- Lp-PLA2 is an enzyme that can assess the amount of inflammation in your arteries due to a build-up of cholesterol.
- hsCRP is a protein produced by the liver when inflammation is present somewhere in your body. It's been used to identify risk for infection or chronic inflammation. This protein tests smaller amounts of CRP in the blood. Researchers have shown that high hsCRP levels can indicate heart attack and stroke risk in apparently healthy individuals.
- ADMA (asymmetric dimethylarginine) and SDMA (symmetric dimethylarginine) are compounds made in your body as proteins are degraded, or broken down. These two markers reduce your body's ability to produce nitric oxide, a molecule that helps maintain the inner lining (endothelium) of the artery wall. If these levels

are elevated, it may indicate endothelial dysfunction and impending damage.

- Oxidized LDL is LDL cholesterol (the "bad" cholesterol) that's been modified by oxidation. Oxidized LDL triggers inflammation, leading to the formation of plaque in arteries, also known as coronary artery disease or atherosclerosis.

- F2-Isoprostanes can cause blood vessels to constrict, which may raise your blood pressure, and promote blood clotting, resulting in a heart attack or stroke. In support of this, F2 Isoprostans may be elevated at the earliest stages of plaque development in your arteries. Research shows that people with high levels of F2-Isoprostanes are thirty times more likely to develop heart disease. This unique marker is measured not by blood but by urine.

- TMAO (trimethylamine N-Oxide) is a byproduct of gut bacteria metabolism. When certain types of bacteria in the gut digest food components found in red meat, eggs, and full-fat dairy products, they release a compound called TMA (trimethylamine), which your liver converts to TMAO. TMAO has been shown to affect how cholesterol is accumulated in tissues, like the artery wall. Abnormally elevated levels of TMAO are associated with increased risk for developing atherosclerotic heart disease, having a heart attack or stroke, and even death.

- OmegaCheck—Omega -3 and Omega-6 are two of the most important types of polyunsaturated fatty acids. Omega-3s help brain and red cell production as well as improve cell membrane health. Our bodies don't make enough omega-3s, so we must get them from the food we eat, such as oily fish and certain plants oils. The most common form of omega-6s come from animal foods in your diet, such as meat and eggs. Arachidonic acid can squelch out the omega-3s and allows for an inflammatory system to be upregulated.

- Microalbumin (Albumin) is a protein that is normally found in your blood and not normally found in your urine. The microalbumin test is able to measure very small amounts of albumin that can leak into the urine. If albumin is in the urine, in even small amounts, this may be indicative of kidney disease or other issues injuring the vessels of your kidneys, such as diabetes, high blood pressure, or autoimmune diseases like lupus.

Have you heard of these markers before? If not, it's high time to start asking. Prevention is the key. These markers are not only important to understand but to have measured in your system. These are indicators that can help you prevent plaque build-up through a chronic inflammatory cascade. If you know the levels and the degree of fire you have in your system, you can often fix it all together, slow it down, and in some cases even reverse it.

Our main goal, of course, is prevention. We wish to provide you with the knowledge you need to prevent heart disease altogether. This is another feather in the hat for freedom—freedom from chronic sickness and disease.

How do we improve these markers? You can improve or fix them by reducing the inflammation in the endothelium, the lining of the artery (which is only one cell thick by the way), with changes in nutrition and lifestyle.

In case you're wondering about the endothelium (I know we're throwing some big words out), here's a little more explanation. The endothelium is the single cell layer that lines every blood vessel in your body. One little tiny cell is designed to protect you from anything leaking across it. This single cell layer is all that's protecting what goes through your bloodstream from getting into your system until it reaches its appropriate place. The appropriate place is the capillaries that are widespread throughout our bodies and allow diffusion of nutrients into tissues to give life to our vital organs. Amazing, isn't it? This inner layer is only *one cell thick*. So how much do you think it would take to damage one cell?

Hardening of the arteries often doesn't show its ugly head until one reaches middle age, let's say around menopause for women and andropause for men.

When the endothelium is damaged, LDL cholesterol can become wedged underneath and then attacked by the immune system. A war begins through the process of oxidation, and fatty plaque can build up.

Our bodies are inherently designed to be well and to fight against sickness and disease. We continue to hit them with so many inflammatory shock waves—sugars, grains, breads, the standard American lifestyle, drugs, alcohol, cigarettes, toxic relationships, and stress—the body becomes inflamed.

So how do we dampen this inflammation?

The number one remedy is awareness. Is your hemoglobin A1C level, or blood sugar, up? Are your triglyceride levels up? Is your blood pressure up? Is your weight up? Each one of these risk factors is an independent risk factor for heart disease. The more risk factors you have, the more the risk. Remember the term *metabolic syndrome*? If we don't look at the risk factors and get them fixed immediately, we're setting ourselves up for the number one killer.

If we start on a plan early by taking all the components of lifestyle seriously, one can avoid, or minimize, the effects of cardiovascular disease. It all begins with understanding inflammation and its causes. Inflammation is the precursor to all chronic sickness and disease, especially heart disease

So let's talk about inflammation for a second. Inflammation is part of the complex biological response of body tissues to harmful stimuli, such as pathogens, damaged cells, or irritants. It's a protective response that involves immune cells. The purpose of inflammation is to eliminate the initial cause of cell injury, clear out cells and tissues damaged from the original insult, and initiate tissue repair.

Inflammation can be classified as either acute or chronic. Acute inflammation is the initial response of the body to harmful stimuli and is achieved by the increased movement of white blood cells from the blood into the injured tissues. This causes heat, redness, swelling, loss of function, and pain or itching

Prolonged inflammation, known as chronic inflammation, leads to a progressive shift in the type of cells present at the site of inflammation and is characterized by simultaneous destruction of the tissue from the inflammatory process. All chronic disease starts as acute inflammation.

Acute inflammation can be characterized by a cut, bruise, broken bone, or tissue damage. It's short term and necessary. A great analogy may be like a fire department crew fighting a fire and then returning to the fire house to clean the engine, hoses, and fire house. The body is equipped to handle "bodily fires" much like this.

On the other hand, chronic inflammation can be characterized by systemic and highly activated inflammatory responses circulating in your bloodstream and going everywhere. These are long term and can last months or years. In this case, the analogy would be like a fire department crew going from fire to fire and having no time to do routine maintenance and cleaning—completely exhausted, overworked, and weak. In this case, the body is totally overwhelmed and can't handle all the "alarm calls" for the many bodily fires.

We've put together a seven-step process for you to employ to prevent heart disease.

1. You must educate yourself.

    Understand what causes heart disease, heart attacks, and strokes. The answer is your lifestyle. The way you live your life every day is what causes arterial inflammation, stiffening of the artery wall, and plaque buildup, which eventually leads to a heart attack of the heart or a heart attack of the brain, also known as a stroke.

Invasive procedures like a double bypass heart surgery or even a placement of a stent don't correct the long-term underlying chronic disease of the arterial system. It's the anti-inflammatory nature of your nutritional plan and the choices you place at the end of your fork that will keep your arterial system healthy. Yes, the most important medical decision you make every day is at the end of your fork.

2. Know your risk factors.

It's not just a simple cholesterol panel that will tell you whether or not you have heart disease. You must do a full panel exam and know all your vital signs. Be passionate about maintaining a healthy body composition. Buy a blood pressure cuff and keep your blood pressure in the normal range. Understand all markers that are biochemical in nature and indicate systemic inflammation, a brewing heart attack, or a stroke. Only you can take the steps to improving your risk factors. Your doctor doesn't have control over your actions at the lunch table or your decision to eat or not eat at a fast food restaurant.

3. It's imperative that you exercise.

We know you can't outrun the fork. Your body will see the toxic nature of food no matter how much you exercise. Exercise is important for keeping the heart healthy and the nature of your heart pumping strong. Exercise is also imperative for depositing minerals in the bones, keeping them strong as well. Exercise also maintains the amount of lean muscle mass you have on your frame. If you don't maintain muscular strength, you'll find yourself weaker than you should be when you're in your 80s and approaching your 90s.

4. Get plenty of adequate rest.

The nature of sleep is vital to the health of the cardiovascular system. A system that's continuously running on overdrive will eventually cause undue damage. When the system doesn't rest, cortisol, epinephrine, and norepinephrine levels rage out of control. Epinephrine and norepinephrine can create abnormal blood pressure readings and cause excessive stress on the heart. The body's natural circadian rhythm will also be out of balance. It's as if the system no longer knows whether it's coming or going. This also leads to problems with hormonal imbalance.

5. Change your diet to a nutritional lifestyle.

We've coined our wellness program, the New American Lifestyle. We know diets don't work. The first three letters of the word *diet* spells die! We have to develop a better relationship with food. We must know that food is the gasoline that runs our engines. If we take in food that has low octane and no nutrition, how is the heart supposed to run like a fine-tuned engine? Changing habits are difficult but imperative in determining the long-term health of the cardiovascular system.

6. Renew your mind.

"As you think, so shall you become." What you have in your mind will get seated in your heart. If your mind is toxic, it will create a toxic environment in your heart. To be completely and totally well, we have to be well in all areas of our lives, including our mind.

7. Start taking the right supplements.

There are a few nutrients you can't go wrong with adding to your daily plan. At the top of the list is EPA and DHA. Our bodies can't make these two omega-3 fatty acids. They must be obtained from the outside. If we don't have enough of these essential fatty acids, our bodies become brittle and rigid. Adding good oil to your system is like changing oil in the engine of your car. This can improve the aging of the vascular system. If the cellular membranes don't have enough EPA and DHA in their phospholipid membranes, they get inflamed, brittle, and stiff, and are more likely to succumb to the inflammatory processes of a heart attack or stroke.

Niacin or vitamin B3 is an important B vitamin that can aid in reducing inflammatory particle sizes and improve good cholesterol numbers. You want to be under the guidance of a physician in adding this nutrient to your protocol to ensure you don't have side effects.

Coenzyme Q10 is another nutrient that's essential for heart health. As we age, our body is unable to make the levels of Coenzyme Q10 they were once able to. Supplementing with Coenzyme Q10 can improve mitochondrial function and energy production. The heart muscle is very rich in mitochondria.

Staying healthy is your responsibility. The bottom line is, we can't depend on physicians, personal trainers, psychiatrists, pastors, or others to keep us healthy. It's a personal responsibility. We must be well educated, and we must make a personal decision to be accountable for our own health. No longer can we depend upon drugs and surgeries to solve the root cause. It's our lifestyle.

It's completely unnecessary to have hundreds and thousands of dollars in medical bills. This can be completely avoided if we take charge, exercise self-control, and take personal action.

Educate yourself, get a thorough workup, understand your inflammatory risk, and do something about it to live a healthy lifestyle. It's fantastic to know that if we get in a medical crisis, we have options available.

These steps will ensure that your life is of *quality* not just *quantity*.

No one is afraid to die—it's the suffering we're fearful of. That can be avoided if we take action.

Feeling Swell

Nutritionally, most inflammation in the body comes from sugar. Sugar lends a byproduct called advanced glycosylated end products. AGEs (no pun intended) make proteins in the body sticky and wreak havoc on that tiny one-celled endothelial lining of the blood vessels. This is why diabetics lose their limbs, their eyes, and their kidneys and little by little kill their blood vessels. They die first and foremost from heart disease.

Thanks to the food pyramid, introduced decades ago, Americans were told to eat six to eight servings of grains per day and eliminate fats. What did that do to body compositions? It began the nationwide onset of obesity. The CDC now predicts that by 2030, across the board, 60 to 100 percent of the population will be either overweight or obese. Do we really have to accept this prediction? We hope not! Certainly not without a fight!

Thinking fat was the problem, the marketplace then drastically replaced fat with sugar. The fat-free craze hit the market. Fake fats, trans fats, and hydrogenated oils replaced mother nature's good fats. *Fat-free cookie, anyone?* Little did we know, taking the fat out was making foods ten times worse. Not looking at the complex carbohydrates as sugars and then altering the fat content in food was causing serious metabolic disruption. Americans were missing the foundational concepts of nutrition.

The standard American diet is inflammatory by design and puts our bodies at risk of heart disease by changing our inflammatory markers: blood pressure, weight, blood sugars, high triglycerides, and low HDL cholesterol.

Tests can measure inflammation, but most people don't get tested and tend to wait until there's a big medical event. Then most go to the doctor, say they don't feel well, and find out the diagnosis is heart disease, when it could've been prevented by being aware, making changes, and staying the course.

Keep in mind that just because you look good on the outside doesn't mean you're healthy on the inside. What you can't see can be grounds for disaster. Just because someone is thin doesn't mean they're not sick. Just because someone has a pretty face does not mean they are free from inflammation and the precursors to heart disease.

The most important course of action is: *don't guess, test!*

If you get tested and don't have someone to explain the results, you probably need to find someone who's been medically trained in understanding the inflammatory pathways and what to do to influence them in the direction of health. If you're offered only pills and no adjustments in lifestyle and nutrition, more than 85 percent of foundational health and wellness has been overlooked. We must address lifestyle if we want to be completely and totally well.

Risk and Remedy Factors

We've spent a lengthy amount of time explaining what heart disease actually is, so by now, you must be wondering what the risk factors are for heart disease. What are the remedies? People who have exaggerated Type-A personalities, clenched-teeth, fight-or-flight surges of adrenaline (commonly manifested as frustration, anger, or hostility) appear to be at a greater risk for developing heart disease. These individuals, although highly productive, tend to have higher blood pressure and even tend to take on habits to create a sense of calm, such as smoking, drinking, alcohol, drugs, and overeating/binge-type behaviors.

These habits are associated with increased incidence of CAD (coronary artery disease).

There are eight major risk factors associated with cardiovascular disease:

1. Abnormal Blood Cholesterol

    Generally speaking, a goal of total cholesterol level of 200 or less is desirable. 200 to 239 is borderline high, while 240 or greater is considered high.

    LDL (bad cholesterol) should be below 100, and HDL (good cholesterol) should be between 40 and 59, with 60 and above even better.

2. Hypertension (High Blood Pressure)

    Normal blood pressure is considered to be 120/80. A reading of 120–139/80–89 is considered to be "prehypertensive." A level of 140–159/90–99 is called stage I hypertension (medical urgency). A level of 160/100 is stage II (medical emergency).

3. Tobacco Use

    Tobacco use of all kinds—smoking, chewing, ingesting nicotine in any form—is directly correlated with cardiovascular disease. There is no "safe" cigarette, cigar, pipe, or any other form of taking in nicotine.

4. Pre-Diabetes (Metabolic Syndrome)

    Pre-diabetes, or metabolic syndrome, is classified as having three of the five markers out of balance. These markers are blood sugar, triglycerides, low HDL, waist greater than thirty-five inches in a female and greater than forty inches in a male (or waist-to-hip ratio greater than 1 in a male or greater than 0.5 in a female), and high blood pressure (any reading greater than 135/85). A normal fasting blood glucose level is 70–99 mg/dl. Fasting blood glucose levels between 100–125 mg/dl on two separate occasions is considered pre-diabetes. Other numbers that need to be looked at and considered are fasting insulin levels great than 5 and Hga1c levels greater than 5.4. The glycomark is also a test that can indicate issues with managing sugars. Triglycerides are high when they are over 150. HDL less than 45 in males and less than 50 in females is a risk factor.

5. Family History

If you have a male blood relative with a history of coronary artery disease prior to age fifty-five or a female blood relative with a coronary artery disease event prior to the age of sixty-five, you may have a genetic link to cardio-vascular disease. Watching what you eat and moving more is something you *can* do to mediate the negative factors of your family medical history.

6. Sedentary Lifestyle

A person should get up and move around for two minutes for every twenty minutes of sitting. Put a little sticky-note on the corner of your computer: *Move!*

A person should engage in at least thirty minutes of moderately intense physical activity at least three days a week. The American Heart Association standard goal is to get 150 minutes of exercise per week. This does not include being active at work. It takes effort to keep your heart muscle strong. We have to challenge and work it. Sitting is regarded as the new smoking. It will take its toll on your heart health if you don't kick the sitting habit.

7. Obesity

Linked to abdominal fat, also called visceral fat, obesity is a major concern. Measure the waist to hip ratio. If it is greater than 1.0 in males and .8 in females, call it obesity. Body fat percentages are also important. Body fat percent goals in men should be between 10 and 20 percent and between 18 and 28 percent in females.

8. Age

Males forty-five years of age and older and females ages fifty-five and older are at greater risk for CAD than those who are younger. If we take better care of ourselves with a healthy lifestyle, our chronological age may not be demonstrated in our physiological age.

Remedies

The American Heart Association provides the following remedies for the above risk factors for CAD:

1. Cholesterol

Cholesterol can be addressed by increasing physical activity, making better nutritional choices, decreasing body fat, managing stress better, controlling diabetes, and stopping use of tobacco products. The medical community is now advancing our approach by using genetic factors that indicate dysfunctional lipid metabolism and sugar metabolism and give insight into how to fix them.

2. Hypertension

To manage blood pressure, genetics may play a role. There are genes that indicate salt sensitivity, caffeine sensitivity, and hypertensive tendencies. We must manage salt, caffeine, and stress. For those who are genetically predisposed to blood pressure issues, their lifestyle must be even tighter in order to avoid the long-term consequence.

Stress is a major factor in controlling blood pressure. When one is under stress, not only is cortisol produced, which alters blood sugar control and contributes to weight gain, but also epinephrine and norepinephrine are produced, the fight or flight hormones. These ratchet up internal tension, leading to high blood pressure, otherwise known as hypertension (high tension).

3. Tobacco Use

Stop using all tobacco products. Period. When it comes to smoking, the only word necessary is *quit*. Smoke and smoke-related behaviors produce carcinogens that are destructive to the vascular system and destroy the cardiovascular system.

4. Pre-Diabetes

Type 2 diabetes is a disease of the affluent. This is a symptom of bad or negligent behavior when we look at its precursors. Since type 2 diabetes is a disease of progression, we can regress it by getting the risk factors that cause it under control. If we are diligent about following a low-glycemic, appropriate calorie, high nutrient dense nutritional plan along with regular exercise, type 2 diabetes would not exist. Education and implementation is the key.

5. Family History

You can't presently change the genes you've been dealt, but you can avoid engaging in "family events" that include bad eating habits, a sedentary lifestyle with no regular exercise, stressful events, and the use of tobacco! Bad habits you now have may have been learned from your family. Unlearn those habits!

You can have your genes tested to evaluate the risk factors you may be predisposed to. Question is, if you know you have a predisposition to diabetes or heart disease, do you have the self-discipline it takes to walk down the path toward fixing it?

6. Obesity

The solution is usually linked to increased physical activity, better nutritional choices, better stress management, and specific physician-supervised programs to decrease body fat. The goal of any weight-loss plan should include the *increase* of muscle mass. We must pay attention to body composition as a whole. We also have to address hormone balance as well. If the thyroid is sick, weight loss can be difficult. If the male and female sex hormone balance is in trouble, weight loss can be difficult. Remember, insulin is a hormone, and when the blood sugar insulin balance isn't in control, weight loss will be difficult.

A great deal of poor physical health is related to bad eating habits—generally too much food or eating foods with very low nutritional benefit, or eating foods without a proper balance of protein, carbohydrates, and healthy fatty acids. In other words, a poor diet. Remember, the first three letters of the word *diet* spell *die*. One of the reasons people don't stick to a diet is they feel like they're going to die after they have been on it for a day or two. That's why we never prescribe diets. Diets don't work. People are individuals, and so are their nutritional needs. We have to follow a nutritional program that has the micronutrients and macronutrients in them to heal and sustain life. Such a nutritional plan lends vitality and quality of life. Weight loss is a side effect of wellness.

For those who are obese or in ill health owing to a poor diet, the main changes to be made are simple. Before spending money on allergy testing or even micronutrient tests, we use an elimination plan in which patients give up:

- breads;
- most grains;

- sugar;
- processed foods;
- fast food;
- gluten;
- soy; and
- dairy.

The plan is simple: eat fresh and raw fruits and vegetables, nuts and seeds, and good clean protein, and drink plenty of water.

Most processed foods have sugars in some form, including both canned and packaged foods.

7. Age

Be grateful you've reached your current age and can make good decisions about increasing the quality of your life as you move forward.

Please note that as shown above, there is something you can do about six of the eight cardiovascular disease factors and their remedies. Which means you can greatly impact 75 percent of the risk factors leading to coronary artery disease and the heart attacks and strokes that can result.

Time for Some More PIES

Physically, let's be honest with ourselves. Is your body carrying a layer of fat that's keeping you from enjoying health? Is this fat a protective armor that keeps you locked into sickness and disease? Is there a root that needs to be discovered and pulled out? At this point, can you identify a key takeaway point from the above discussion and put together an action step to get physical improvement?

Intellectually, the first fact to keep in mind is that you have a tremendous amount of control over the health of your heart. You're not destined to be sick; you're designed to be well, and you are even equipped to recover from many setbacks—even self-induced ones. Knowledge is power, and we can help you put that knowledge into a life-changing plan to reclaim your health. What will you do with this new knowledge?

Emotionally, it's okay not to enjoy a discussion of deadly disease. But channel the energy of fear into positive action. And remember that facts are your friend, because they ultimately can eliminate fear and dread. Once you know the facts, there's no guilt, no shame, only consequences of continual behavior and action. We understand that emotions can be fickle and ever-changing. However, let's act on facts! Right actions must lead emotions. Don't worry, the emotions will quickly follow and line up. What action will you now take to overcome negative emotion?

Spiritually, focus on your vision for life. Who do you serve? Who is your master? Is it God, food, alcohol, or other health-destroying behaviors? Is your spiritual life dead? Are you searching for answers? If you don't know, then perhaps it's time to search for what drives you, spiritually. Don't be a victim of spiritual death, it will eventually lead to chronic sickness and disease. Is there a sense of life and hope boiling inside you right now? We sure hope so!

Eliminate fear with facts and action. After all, wouldn't you rather be in control of your future?

6

Dodging Diabetes

TYPE 2 DIABETES IS MORE A SYMPTOM THAN A DISEASE. WHEN I (Michele) started my medical residency, there were only a few type 2 diabetic medications. We voraciously memorized the laundry lists of side effects and interactions, times of day to take them, and monthly costs at the pharmacy so we could advise our patients.

Now, there are at least thirty different types of medication for type 2 diabetes, and the disease is on the rise. We can't memorize them all anymore. Instead, we go to our phones to display our fancy pharmacopias to find the answers. If we know the root causes, then why are we throwing pills at the problem?

This isn't okay and shouldn't be considered normal. Type 2 diabetes is almost always avoidable. A type 2 diabetic shouldn't accept this lifelong expensive, health-destroying, sentence when he or she can do something about it.

Insulin is just a band-aid on a wound. It does nothing to eradicate the cause of the wound. Sugar is at the root of type 2 diabetes. There's a long physiologic process that happens in the onset of type 2 diabetes. Taking in excess sugar causes a state of insulin resistance and blood sugar mismanagement. It's as if the locks and keys of blood sugar and insulin don't fit. The locks become rusty and the body gets confused.

Often this stage begins five to ten years before the diagnosis of type 2 diabetes. There is a class of medications that are used only in the type 2 diabetic. These medications are used to manage all the broken pathways of blood sugar mismanagement in the body, before the pancreas wears completely out and we have to add insulin.

In order to eradicate the retinopathy, the nephropathy, neuropathy, the cutting off of limbs, and the heart disease of a diabetic, we have to get to the cause. Of course medications are often necessary when we have a disease that's out of control. What we must do is become wise to the cause of the disease and do something about it before it ever gets started.

Based on our experience, most diabetics don't know they have to give up sugar. Many have never been told. Refined sugar should never be part of the lifestyle of a diabetic. Doctors need to let patients know that sugar is poison.

Many clinicians and dieticians recommend counting carbohydrates and actually recommend certain increases in insulin to help balance the body's inability to manage the sugar load. A surprising number in the medical community are allowing type 2 diabetes to worsen by suggesting band aids instead of getting to the root. If sugar is the cause, it must be addressed. Instead of bringing the cause of the disease to light, they're treating symptoms.

Are You a Diabetic?

The question is more complicated than you might think. If you are diagnosed with type 2 diabetes, don't make any changes to your medications without consulting a doctor. And if your doctor has never looked you in the eye and told you exactly what to do to get better—or told you to get off medications—it might be time to find a new doctor.

So why is this question complicated?

Once you are given the diagnosis of diabetes, you're identified by that diagnosis. That diagnosis never goes away in your medical chart. Even if you change your biomarkers and all the markers of metabolic syndrome and insulin resistance markers that classified you as a risk for diabetes, the diagnosis never goes away.

If you change your lifestyle and normalize your markers for diabetes, you're still considered a diabetic by your health insurance company. Does this mean the battle isn't worth it? Of course not! Health is its own reward. You can enjoy every day.

Knowledge is power. If we know what to do to prevent the disease, why would we not choose to live in accordance with a life free from the illness? Is it an internal disobedience? Is it rebellion? Is it a cop-out, like saying, "My parents had diabetes, so I will have it too?"

Most diabetics die from heart disease and the complications from diabetes. It's a road of unnecessary suffering. Living a healthy lifestyle is difficult. Living a life with the challenges of type 2 diabetes is much more difficult, frightening, and painful.

If you're not a diabetic, it's almost a certainty that you can avoid that label for the rest of your life. It's worth the fight to avoid being labeled a diabetic—another fact that too few medical professionals proclaim. Once you have this label, so many aspects of your life will be affected.

In addition to the mental and emotional strain of the condition, your life insurance and health insurance rates will skyrocket. Is this needless spending? Of course it is! So now we ask, if you decide to change and live a life empowered by nutrition and a healthy lifestyle, are you needlessly spending money? Obviously, the answer is no. Let's spend that money elsewhere and on nutrition that gives and brings life.

In this life, we have to pick our pleasures carefully. In today's society, most people pick food.

Your Best Friend

Food is some people's only high point of the day. It's easy to get trapped on the vicious cookie cycle, seeking comfort from food.

Snacks are some people's best friend. People betray you, but a bag of Oreos won't. A bag of chips will do exactly what you want it to do—it will love you . . . until it kills you.

Deep down, comfort food is a control mechanism. When someone loses control of their life—their weight, their marriage, their finances, their home, their kids—they naturally want some predictability and control. They go in search of comfort. Often, the comforter is food. After all, this is what we learned as children.

It's difficult to address the concept of food providing emotional comfort, but it's a fact we all deal with at some level. Many of the sugars that drive type 2 diabetes stimulate the same dopamine receptors in the brain that cocaine does. They cause dopamine, the "happy hormone," to generate in the body, which makes people feel good. But while the feeling is short lived, the addiction is real.

Do You Feel the Resistance?

If the thought of giving up, or greatly reducing, your favorite comfort food makes you sad, fearful, or angry, please stay with us.

We understand there are actual withdrawal symptoms—physical, intellectual, and emotional. You can't imagine feeling so good that you won't even miss a certain drug—or food. Here's a reminder to trust us. There is a way to live, and a way to feel, that so transcends pizza, or ice cream, that you'll wonder how those foods ever controlled you. This might seem impossible to imagine, but it's true.

If you're surrounded by others struggling with diabetes, including family members, this disease might seem inevitable, but it's not.

Memo to Doctors

Type 2 diabetes should not exist to the degree it does today, with increasing numbers of medications and increasing cases of the disease. Something is wrong. It's wrong at the root, wrong at the core.

Doctors take an oath to do no harm, but diabetic education isn't just falling short, it's causing harm. Patients aren't taught to get off sugar, they're instead taught to manage it with medications. Sure, we learn about carb counting and adding insulin, but what about minimizing carbohydrates, increasing exercise (whose action is more powerful on lowering blood sugar than insulin), and minimizing the use of unnecessary medications? Shouldn't that be the goal?

When someone withholds truth that could heal a patient or prevent a disease, isn't that causing harm? Isn't that allowing a person to partake in slow, self-inflicted, uneducated suicide? In a sense, it's murderous behavior. Of course, this is an eye-opening perspective.

Patients must make their own decisions. They rely on medical professionals to provide facts and answers. You can lead a horse to water, but you can't make him drink. We must place emphasis on the facts that prevention, reversal, and cure lie in the hands of the patient. The degree that one chooses to care for one's health and longevity will be the degree to which one reaps the reward. No guilt, only consequences.

Doctors take so much blame for their patients' health. *I went to six doctors and nobody could fix me. My doctor put me on these medicines that gave me such terrible side effects. My doctor told me I could eat sugar, I just have to take more medicine.* Sound familiar?

Doctors and clinicians can help by providing the right diagnosis, guidance, and tools for healing, but it's ultimately up to the individual to take the steps. These steps aren't just short-lived steps that last for a few days or a few months. These steps must be followed for the rest of your life.

No Matter Your Weight

Did you know that you can be skinny and still be fat? Just because you're thin doesn't mean you're healthy. There's a term called *sarcopenic obesity* (skinny fat). You can never judge a book by its cover. That's why it's so important to understand your body composition and not be focused on scale weight. There are many slim patients with 45 percent body fat. Remember, the healthy body fat range for women is 18 to 28 percent, and for men it is 10 to 18 percent.

Some people's frames can carry fat more discretely. They look somewhat normal but are really puffy marshmallows. This is a medical condition defined as the presence of low muscle mass and either low muscle strength or low physical performance. When this is accompanied by a high fat mass, we have the aforementioned condition of sarcopenic obesity. This is why "body composition" is a vital measurement. Many doctors rely on body mass index (BMI), but this measure is crude and doesn't reveal lean mass, fat mass, and intracellular and extracellular water. And it doesn't show someone's basal metabolic rate.

Additionally, BMI doesn't account for individuals with increased bone mass, increased muscle mass, or increased height. In these individuals, the BMI can appear to show morbid obesity. The body composition analysis is an accurate way of making choices, so the applied nutritional and exercise protocol isn't burning off muscle mass as fuel and cellular health is improving. If we're working hard to live a healthy life, we want to have a viable measure that indicates accurate progress.

When I (Michele) speak to groups of colleagues, athletes, or individuals wanting to better their health, I will often ask, "How many of you know what your basal metabolic rate is? How many of you know what your body composition is made up of?"

Maybe one or two out of a hundred generally raise their hands. We can't change what we don't know. How are physicians and clinicians supposed to educate on improving body composition and the components of health if they haven't mastered it in their own lives?

It's Really Simple

Over the years, we've taken plenty of criticism from people who say our approach to wellness is "overly simplistic." We take that as a compliment.

Ironically, the people who tell us our recommendations are too simple can't actually do it themselves. And, sadly, their health isn't what it could be.

Everyone is looking for some complex secret, but wellness is really about the basics. Now, as you've probably figured out already, making simple changes isn't simple. But keep this in mind: your body was designed for wellness. Treat your body right—along with your intellect, emotions, and heart—and your overall health will improve.

One challenge in creating a wellness lifestyle, especially when it comes to type 2 diabetes, is how often we're bombarded with media messages about unhealthy food. Our senses are constantly indulged with images of sweet treats, biggie sized drinks, and magnitudes of unhealthy choices.

Some of the most influential people in the world, including professional athletes, agree to advertise sugary cereals, soft drinks, and so-called energy drinks. All of which can contribute to the type 2 diabetes epidemic. Sadly, this epidemic isn't just among adults anymore, but is spilling over into our young people. Children are becoming afflicted with this sugar-based disease.

As athletes ourselves, we can tell you that you'll rarely see those elite spokespersons actually consuming the unhealthy foods and drinks they tout in advertisements.

Many former athletes who are now diabetic have come through our office. They gave up daily exercise and lost control over their nutrition. They weren't completely aware of the consequences, so how could they count the cost? Again, health is simple. Making the change can be difficult. But it's worth it.

A quick diet won't change the long-term trajectory of your life. Neither will a pill. You can't outrun what you put on the end of your fork. You can't burn off poison. What has to happen is a change in the heart that adopts a long-term lifestyle change including appropriate nutrition and exercise.

The Whole-Being Shift

Yes, we need to clean out our refrigerator and kitchen cabinet, but that's not enough. We need to open up our hearts and clean out our emotional cabinets with all the excess baggage in order to move toward freedom.

To use another analogy, it's hard work to go into a garden and pull up all the weeds. When you pull up the weeds, other stuff (more roots and shoots) sometimes appears. When you pull on a root, FRAUDS sometimes pop up—fear, resentment, anger, unforgiveness, disappointment, and shame. In the moment, it might be painful to deal with, but in the end you'll have a wonderful garden with new growth. A free heart is a happy heart—one that can make healthy choices for a life filled with vitality.

To truly get well—physically, intellectually, emotionally, spiritually—you have to be willing to go to the root. If you're willing to go there, you *will* get better.

You will get better. The choice is up to you. No guilt, only consequences.

The following is a classic example of an individual who tries desperately to outrun/out-exercise the fork. This person is an elite cyclist who's a very vocal proponent for exercise. At age fifty-seven, she exercises up to two hours a day. Her body composition by measure is sarcopenic obese. She is thin, and her attitude exudes health. She encourages everyone to eat anything they want, just do more exercise and work it off. Her theory is exercise is all you need to be healthy. Sounds great, right? But her blood pressure is very high (a state of high tension also known as hypertension), she has atrial fibrillation (an abnormal heart rhythm), her bones demonstrate osteoporosis (which means her bones are thin and relatively weak). Osteoporosis can be caused by poor nutrition, over-exercise, and hormone imbalance.

She's rebellious with food—a food junkie with a high carbohydrate diet. Her bones are rotting, her heart is stressed with high blood pressure, and her blood sugar is high, but she thinks she's healthy because she's thin. This is a good example of judging a book by its cover. However, just because you're thin doesn't mean you're healthy.

It's not normal to have high blood pressure, it's not normal to have high blood sugar, it's not normal to have osteoporosis. It's not normal to be sarcopenic obese. You can be skinny, but if you have a protruding belly, that's a warning sign. Your body may be saying, *I'm starving to death.* Many times it's the symbol of the body looking for something you aren't giving it—not only nutritionally, but perhaps some peace, love, and rest. There's a disruption in total balance that needs to be addressed.

The question is, do you believe disease is "normal" for you?

Changing Normal

Our *normal* has now become abnormal, and the *abnormal* has now become normal. This generation is the first generation with more overweight and sick people than well people. In today's America, if you're fit and healthy with a normal body composition, you're radically different.

Patients who make healthy changes often receive very interesting comments from friends and family. People will almost never tell you that you're too fat, but how many times have you heard someone comment when you begin to get your life under control and lose the unnecessary weight, "You look so skinny. Are you okay? Are you sure you are not sick?"

We don't know why there's not more positive pressure from our society and the medical community to be well. We understand that some unhealthy people are uncomfortable when others make healthy change. But why wouldn't the medical community shout from the rooftops, *Type 2 diabetes is a man-made disease!*

Diabetes is a multi-billion dollar business. We're not anti-pharmaceuticals—in many cases, medications are lifesavers. We believe in avoiding disease at all costs. Why spend your hard-earned money on pills and medical bills when you don't have to?

Five Symptoms That Lead to Diabetes

The big diabetes buzzwords these days are *pre-diabetes, metabolic syndrome, syndrome X,* and *insulin resistance.* These are all precursors to the horrible disease.

With nutrition and exercise, you can control your cholesterol, triglycerides, blood pressure, HgA1c, fasting insulin levels, and blood sugar levels. Keeping these markers in line will stave off pre-diabetes, metabolic syndrome, syndrome X, insulin resistance, and type 2 diabetes.

If you have any of the following symptoms, you should have your biomarkers for diabetes checked.

1. At any age, if you are overweight, you may be at risk. Visceral fat (fat around your midsection) has been shown to carry a higher risk. An increased waist-to-hip ratio is not a good thing—it means more fat around the middle. For every pound you're overweight, it puts ten pounds pressing down on your joints. If you're twenty pounds overweight, multiply that by ten. That is two hundred extra pounds you're lugging around. If we don't get weight under control, how are we going to feel at the end of the day? Weight stresses the heart, stresses the bones, and even stresses the endocrine system and hormone balance.

2. Sitting too much is a risk factor. Sitting has been called "the new smoking." Exercise is second only to nutrition as an important way to control your risk and has been shown to be more powerful than insulin in lowering blood sugars. Inactivity leads to muscle loss and a lower basal metabolic rate. This means you burn less calories per day and more calories may be stored as fat. When you begin to lose muscle, you begin to get weak. When you feel weak, you're more inclined to eat than you are to exercise.

3. Elevated blood pressure is telling you that your body is under too much tension. (It's called *hypertension* after all, meaning a state of high tension.) Even though the JNC 8 (Joint National Committee Guideline for the management of blood pressure) has changed the standards on blood pressure control, make sure you talk to your doctor to ensure your blood pressure isn't harming your health. High blood pressure is a silent killer because it pounds away at your kidneys, brain, eyes, and nerves. It's called the silent killer because it can't be felt and often goes undiagnosed.

4. If you have high blood lipids (also known as blood fats-cholesterol), either triglycerides or cholesterol (LDL), you are likely at risk. Triglycerides (triglycerides greater than 150 mg/dl) have moved to the front of the line as a marker for metabolic syndrome and pre-diabetes. Low HDL cholesterol is also a risk factor. This number should be greater than 45 mg/dl in men and more than 50 mg/dl in women. Non-HDL cholesterol total and cholesterol particle size should also be considered.

5. Check your family history for risk factors, but don't let your genes be an excuse to give in to diabetes. This should motivate you even more to stop the madness and get ahold of your lifestyle right away. In today's times, we know the power of nutrigenetics and nutrigenomics, which is the scientific study of the interaction of genes on the environment and of nutrition on gene expression, especially with regards to the prevention or treatment of disease. Just because you're born with a predisposition toward type 2 diabetes doesn't mean you need to develop it.

Talk to your doctor about your biomarkers of risk and have your full fasting blood panel, HgA1c, fasting insulin, fasting blood lipid panel, body composition, and blood pressure checked as soon as possible. You may want to go one step beyond and consider genetic testing for your health, metabolic, and exercise profile, which can be used to customize a nutrition and exercise protocol uniquely for you.

Knowledge is power.

Type 2 diabetes is a man-made disease. We don't have to be victims and resign ourselves to a future tied to pills and ills. The good news about this bad news disease is that you can avoid it. If you've been diagnosed with it or want to prevent it from getting its grips on you, find a physician or clinician who can become an accountability partner for your health and has the knowledge and experience to help you change your lifestyle for the better.

Time for PIES

You know the drill. It's time to invest in introspection.

Physically, let's face some truth. Are you avoiding some facts about your physical health? Do you know your body composition? Do you know your basal metabolic rate? Do you know your risk factors? Have you had your biomarkers of inflammation evaluated and explained? Do you know if you're truly healthy or just *not sick?*

Do you know if you fall into the "pre-diabetic/metabolic syndrome" classification?

If the answer to any of the above questions is no, it's time to get busy and find a physician/clinician that can get you started down the path to total health and wellness.

Intellectually, have you bought into the new, unhealthy, normal? Have you resigned yourself to being overweight, out of shape, and (unconsciously) headed toward disease?

Emotionally, have you connected your emotional life with food in any way? We'll discuss this in a later chapter, but all we ask is you begin to recognize the connections.

Spiritually, how about investing in your spiritual life with daily positivity statements? "I'm stress-free and at peace," "I live a continual and intentional life of wellness, while voiding unhealthy food, activities, situations, and people."

7

The War on Cancer

THE MEDICAL COMMUNITY BEGAN A WAR ON CANCER MORE than forty years ago.

Are we learning more about this disease of dread? Yes. Is research helping? Definitely. But we're still not winning the war on cancer.

What Is Cancer?

Cancer is the overproliferation of cells, driven in an abnormal way, to become something they're not designed to be. A cancer is a malignant growth or tumor resulting from the division of tumor cells. Left uncontrolled, these tumor cells can invade nearby tissues. These cells can then spread to other parts of the body through the lymph system or bloodstream. When a person's immune system is strong, the cancer cells being produced are destroyed and prevented from multiplying and forming tumors. When a person has cancer, it indicates the person has multiple nutritional deficiencies and potential toxicities. These toxicities can be genetic, environmental, food-related, and lifestyle-driven. The standard American diet is toxic to the core. Much research is lending itself to the hazards of the food pyramid, fast-food living, and the on–the-run lifestyles our nation has adopted.

Johns Hopkins University Medical Center recently posed an article on sugar's effect on cancer formation. Sugar is one of the root causes of inflammatory disease. Sugar produces advanced glycosylated end products, or AGEs, and these end products are at the root of inflammation, the acceleration of chronic disease, and the development of cancer.

Let's take a look at how glycosylated end products work. AGEs affect nearly every type of cell and molecule in the body and are thought to be one factor in aging and some cancers. They're also believed to play a causative role in the vascular complications of type 2 diabetes mellitus.

Under certain pathologic conditions, such as oxidative stress (rapid rusting) due to high blood sugar in individuals with metabolic syndrome, insulin resistance, diabetes, and or high cholesterol, AGE formation can be increased beyond normal levels. AGEs are now known to play a role as proinflammatory mediators to other chronic disease, which can turn on cell proliferation and run you down the road of cancer.

The animal and human evidence shows that when significant amounts of dietary advanced glycosylated end products are absorbed, AGEs contribute to the body's burden of AGE (inflammation) and are associated with diseases such as heart disease, kidney disease, and ultimately cancer.

AGEs have a range of pathological effects:
Increased blood vessel permeability, or leaky blood vessels.
- Increased blood vessel stiffness. The life is in the blood. If the vessels are stiff, how does good nutrition ensue?
- Inhibition of blood vessel health by damaging the endothelium.
- Increasing the stickiness of inherent proteins, leading to disease and degeneration.

- AGEs bind cells and tissues—in other words, they over-activate the immune system and genetic responses to induce the secretion of a variety of inflammatory proteins that set you up for the development of cancer.

Good nutrition is at the root of the solution. If sugar drives AGE, certainly eliminating it or minimizing it leads to the solution.

The semi-ketogenic, low-glycemic, low sugar load and short intermittent fasting nutrition protocols have now become a way to aid in the treatment of cancer. Sugar is a cancer-feeder. Cutting off sugar cuts off one important food supply to the cancer cells. Sugar alternatives are stevia, truvia, and xylitol, but these should only be consumed in very small amounts. High sugar diets cause release of the hormone insulin. High levels of insulin create a cell receptor resistance. Receptors essentially rust and become ineffective in their ability to transport sugar effectively, increasing the production of AGEs. We must aim for the proper sugar/insulin balance.

When you suppress insulin and learn how to keep it controlled through appropriate nutrition, you allow the body to shift gears into a more metabolically efficient state. In a semi-ketogenic state, insulin is suppressed and the body starts to clean itself up and can more effectively digest unhealthy cells, instead of allowing them to proliferate and keep the cancer fire burning.

Because cancer is an inflammatory disease of cells gone awry, the root causes a large percentage of the time are poor nutrition and lifestyle. You can be tested to know the genes you were given at conception—and you can test for genetic vulnerabilities for certain types of cancer. But we also know how lifestyle influences genes through nutrigenomics—the influence of environment and nutrition on genes. Just because you were born with certain genes (like the P53 genes, BRAC 1 and BRAC 2, or the cystic fibrosis gene, which is not a cancer gene) doesn't mean those genes necessarily have to become active and move in the direction of cancer.

Lifestyle can control much of the outcome. You can control your lifestyle. In fact, science is finding nutrition can control up to 85 percent of your long-term outcome by adhering to a clean nutritional protocol and minimizing chronic inflammation.

Don't Sugar Coat the Issue

Did you know that many people, probably including us, have cancer cells in their body? But most of those cells die. Our bodies fight this war all day every day. The big question is, what makes cell proliferation move in a bad direction? The answer is the environment becomes vulnerable when DNA is altered, and then cells become susceptible to inflammation, and the acceleration of cell proliferation goes in the wrong direction.

The key to avoiding and minimizing cancer is reducing inflammation. Cancer, in the end, is an inflammatory disease. We must begin to change the environment to decrease the incidence of cancer becoming a reality. Lifestyle is at the root. We must change our habits and understanding of nutrition.

Cancer cells thrive in a high sugar environment. But what causes cell death, including the death of cancerous cells? Apoptosis. A number of biochemical events lead to characteristic cell changes (morphology) and death. These changes are usually recognized by the body's defense mechanism and the process of cell death ensues. When cancer cells are out of control, apoptosis doesn't take place at a normal rate. It's as if the body can't see the abnormal cell changes taking place and the cancer cells are then allowed to proliferate and make more of their kind.

A plant-based nutritional environment, semi-ketogenic protocol, allows the body's natural defenses to be cancer resistant. The body's natural defense systems are sharpened, more in tune, and able to get rid of unhealthy cells when supported by a plant-based nutritional environment. Mother Nature provides the right blend of protein, carbohydrates, and fats with the important essential micronutrient ratio the body needs to care for and repair itself and defend against disease.

The problem is, we aren't eating what Mother Nature provides. We have succumbed to unnatural eating habits, including excessive amounts of processed, packaged, sugar-laden foods. Our bodies are nutrient-devoid, sugar-rich, and acidic. Our internal environments are perfect for the development of cancer.

When we adhere to a nutritional plan made up of 80 percent fresh and raw fruits and vegetables with nuts and seeds, this helps put the body into an alkaline environment. About 20 percent of the food we eat can be cooked legumes if there's no allergy or food sensitivity. Fresh and raw fruits and vegetables provide live enzymes that are easily absorbed and aid cellular health.

If we're eating boxed, packaged, processed, sugary, food, not only are we not getting enzymes, we're getting very little micronutrient (vitamin and mineral) nutrition, and we're absorbing and producing massive amounts of AGEs. Keep in mind, when you cook vegetables, the enzymes are destroyed at a temperature of 104 degrees Fahrenheit (40 degrees Celsius). Cooking, however, is necessary for certain health conditions.

When grains are consumed, they're broken down by our bodies into sugar. Our grain-based, standard American diet has led us down the path of sickness and disease. We're not going to laboriously discuss the negative effects of grains on the system, as there are many high-quality resources available, such as the books *Grain Brain* and *Wheat Belly*, to help you wrap your brain around the subject.

Our point here is that processed, packaged, GMO-containing grains have massive health-destroying potential, and their end product in the body is sugar. To say it plainly, avoid sugar and processed, refined, grains. As we discussed in the previous chapter on diabetes, these are poison.

We also recommend you avoid eating excessive meat and animal protein. Meat protein is difficult to digest and requires a lot of digestive enzymes. Undigested meat remaining in the intestines becomes putrefied and leads to more toxic buildup. Eventually, the lining of the gut becomes weak and sets the whole system up for an inflammatory disaster.

Cancer cell walls have a tough protein covering. When we refrain from eating meat or eat less meat, it frees up more enzymes to attack the protein walls of cancer cells and allows the body's killer cells to destroy the cancer cells. Meat and animal products are high in saturated fats that can cause some systems havoc when consumed in excess.

Meat and animal products are also responsible for the production of arachidonic acid. When arachidonic acid goes unbalanced with an inappropriate omega-3 ratio, this leaves a system in a state of inflammation. Arachidonic acid is an omega 6. Our nutritional protocols should be balanced one to one—omega 6 to omega 3, but the standard American diet lends a ratio of twenty to one. Cells don't stand a chance when this ratio becomes obscured. Cell membrane health declines, cell to cell communication is altered, and then the environment becomes perfect for the generation of cancer.

Cancer cells thrive in an acid environment. A meat-based diet is acidic, so it's best to eat fish and a little chicken rather than beef or pork. Meat also contains livestock antibiotics, growth hormones, and, worst case scenario, parasites, which can be present if meat isn't properly packaged, stored, or cooked. All of which are harmful, especially to people with cancer and those trying to avoid it.

Be cautious with the overconsumption of dairy. Milk and milk proteins cause the body to produce mucus, especially in the gastrointestinal (gut) tract. Cancer feeds on mucus. By cutting off milk and substituting with unsweetened almond or coconut milk, you starve the cancer cells of yet another nutrient. Many systems lose their ability to digest the milk protein lactose by losing the ability to produce the enzyme lactase. There's also a very high percentage of the population that has an allergy to casein and other milk-related proteins. We've personally observed this through testing in 80 percent of our six thousand–plus patients.

Choose your nutrition wisely. It can lend to health or it can lend to sickness and disease. Nutritional choices can accelerate or decelerate cancer cell production. Isn't it better to avoid a disease than to have to respond to it?

Risk Factors

Of course, the number one risk factor for cancer is your family history, or your genome—your genetic metabolic and health profile. You're born with a genome that's specific to you. Your lifestyle influences your genome every day. You may be born with a certain genome or risk factor for cancer, but that doesn't mean you have to develop cancer.

Age is another risk factor. For every day you grow older, your cells undergo change. Some die, some stay the same, and others undergo morphologic change. Most often our body's healing machinery prevents cells from becoming cancerous. As you age, that machinery weakens.

Just like you can't change your genes, you can't change your age either. What you can do is change the risk factors you have control over. We now know you can influence your genes by how you live. You may be born with a predisposition for certain types of cancer, but you don't have to add fuel to the fire by turning these present, yet inactive, genes on. The better you take care of yourself all the days of your life, the less likely you will be to age and rust at a rapid rate.

Yes, some people smoke and drink for eighty years and live to over one hundred years without any major medical issues. Genetically, they carry strengths that can withstand the oxidative stress of time and lifestyle. Others are born with oxidative stress weakness, so they show up with diseases due to the damages of oxidative stress, whether it's nutrition, smoking, or alcohol.

Please hear us. Genetics don't necessarily dictate your future. You have more control than you think, and if that's the only takeaway you receive from this book, that's a big win for us and especially for you and your family.

Think of genetics like a card game—everyone is dealt a different set of cards. Those with winning hands sometimes squander the advantage, and those with less favorable hands can make the best of their cards and emerge victorious.

Inflammation is a risk factor and can potentiate the earlier onset of cancer. Cancer has inflammation at its root. Similar to heart disease and diabetes, cancer sometimes results from the barrage of the standard American diet, cigarettes, alcohol, drugs, and other derogatory behaviors.

These negative behaviors can accelerate the genomic expression of what you've inherited and speed the onset of cancer. Inflammation is the precursor to all chronic sickness and disease. When a cell becomes sick or denatured, it's an inflammatory reaction. When we expose our cells to substrates or substances that induce inflammation, cancer can occur at a quicker rate. The more poison in the body, the more the body has to detoxify the elements.

The inability to detoxify is another risk factor. When a person can't eliminate toxins, the toxins dominate the body systems and break down the repair and apoptotic machinery. The body then becomes toxic. These toxins are stored and become persistent pollutants. This toxic environment promotes DNA damage on the cellular level, which is the first step toward mutagenic and carcinogenic activity. DNA damage begins to lead to abnormal cell proliferation. Now cell turnover has gone in the wrong direction, and a tumor is born.

Our bodies were designed to identify and excrete toxins that come in through the air we breathe, the food we eat, and the drinks we consume. We are not garbage cans. We were made to be clean, get clean, and stay clean—in every facet of our being. We must care for our human temples diligently and treat them with respect and good self-care.

Toxic Thoughts and Emotions

We know toxic food, air, and water can cause cancer. That's an established scientific fact.

But we can also point to the work of Dr. Amen regarding changing your brain and changing your life. He speaks to the ANTs, or automatic negative thoughts, that inhabit your mind. His work proves that negative thoughts and emotions affect our physical health. Ask any physician if stress affects our bodies, and the answer will be yes.

Ask yourself if you tangibly feel the impact of fear, anger, unforgiveness, disappointment, and shame in your body. The ongoing effect of these FRAUDS is like emotional cancer. It's not always what you eat, but what eats you.

Medically speaking, thoughts and emotions produce chemicals in our bodies. They drive blood pressure, heart rate, blood sugar, and many other vital signs.

Because we want you to be well in every area of your life, we'd be doing you a disservice if we didn't mention the difference healthy emotions can make when it comes to defeating cancer, avoiding cancer, and living well.

As you're learning, the four facets of our being are all inter-connected and were intended to live in four-part harmony. You already know, on a personal level, the effect emotions and thoughts can have on your resolve and your choices.

The same way you're now evaluating the foods and drinks you consume, evaluate the thoughts and emotions you choose. Be picky about what you put into your heart and soul—as well as your physical temple.

Winning the Battle

We've had patients with lymphoma who've won the war on cancer with good nutrition and exercise—along with megadoses of faith and hope. Now they're on track to stay healthy and more likely to fight off cancer cells.

Once again, let us remind you: our bodies are inherently designed to be well. You can destroy that programming by living a reckless life or you can help it function smoothly by living in accordance with the laws of nature and choosing a healthy lifestyle.

Eight Tips for Kicking Cancer's Butt

Since cancer is a form of inflammation, listed below are some tips to help you take control of inflammation. Remember, all chronic sickness and disease starts with inflammation. Often, the first outward sign of inflammation is excess weight. In our practice, we don't focus on weight because effective weight loss is a side effect of a healthy lifestyle.

1. Conduct one to two days per week of intermittent fasting.

These fasting periods can range from eighteen to twenty-four hours. Don't worry; it's not that bad. Basically, you'll eat your dinner at a normal time, say six o'clock p.m. You won't eat again until around noon the next day. You can have your coffee or water, of course, but don't eat food.

This will allow your body to rest, recover, rebuild, and reset. We've performed blood testing on ourselves to confirm the efficacy of fasting. Based upon our numerous tests, we've seen insulin fall, which leads to fat burning, and we've witnessed the elevation of IGF-1, which equates to muscle building.

2. Eat vegan for two consecutive days.

Give your body a break from all meat sources. A diet high in meat products can be very acidic. These consecutive vegan days will re-alkalize your system. This can work extremely well regarding full-body cleansing and detoxification.

3. Conduct a five-day ketosis cycle.

During this five-day period, you'll eat roughly 70 percent quality fat, 20 percent protein, and 10 percent carbohydrates. This cycle actually works quite well when following or preceding the vegan days.

Make sure not to overdo it in terms of caloric load. Focus on monounsaturated fats and some polyunsaturated fats. Eat no more during these days than two hundred to four hundred calories above your basal metabolic rate. Your basal metabolic rate can be calculated by plugging in your personal numbers online to the easily found Harris-Benedict equation.

4. Drink a shake in the evening.

In this instance, a shake is consumed in the evening instead of a chewed meal. This will give the stomach a break in digestion prior to going to sleep. One of the greatest mistakes people make is to overeat in the evening. This not only disturbs sleep but impairs digestion and can cause excess fat gain.

Make sure to include the following in the shake: quality protein, powdered or actual greens, full fat unsweetened nut or coconut milk, and no more than one cup of a low-glycemic fruit.

5. Practice the "three-bite rule" on desserts.

Let's face it; desserts are present during celebrations. Rather than feeling left out and dealing with issues of deprivation, go ahead and have a bite. Actually, have three. This "three-bite rule" will give you the taste you may temporarily desire and also the enjoyment of the event with family and friends.

6. Limit alcohol to one glass, only two days a week.

Alcohol is also sometimes a part of celebrations. It's also very cultural. Absent total abstinence, this tip will ensure inclusion as well as avoidance of alcohol dependency.

We recommend using this tip during the weekends, allowing one to indulge with one to two glasses of alcohol or even a couple of beers. It's important to note that alcohol does contain calories—one gram of alcohol is seven calories. Be careful, though; alcohol can cause blood sugar crashes, resulting in cravings for sugary and inflammatory foods.

Sugar is present in alcohol as ethanol. Alcohol is toxic. How else would it have such mind-altering and addictive potential? It also requires specific enzymes for its detoxification. If this enzyme isn't present in adequate amounts to meet the consumption, toxicity ensues. Alcoholics put themselves at risk for developing hepatocellular carcinoma. We must mention, however, that if you've already had cancer or currently have that diagnosis, you should avoid or severely limit alcohol or any other known toxins.

It's wise to consume 200 mg of glutathione for each day you consume alcohol. Glutathione is the body's chief antioxidant and is depleted with routine alcohol ingestion.

7. Drink a large glass of water before and during large feasts.

By consuming a large glass of water prior to eating, the stomach will already have a good section filled. This will prevent, and even slow, the propensity to overeat. Additionally, while eating the meal, water can be consumed between bites. This often forgotten tip can substantially reduce food overloading.

Drink plenty of water all day as your mainstay beverage. Our bodies are 60 percent water. They don't function and detoxify as effectively if the hydration status is a quart low.

8. Chew slowly until solid food becomes soup.

Chewing aids in digestion, which actually begins in the mouth. More complex digestion begins in the stomach and small intestine, and completion ends in the large intestine.

Many times, especially in today's society, people are chewing too little and eating too quickly. This leads to many digestive issues, including reflux. When we chew food more thoroughly, the stomach is allowed to fill at a proper pace. In turn, this allows the brain to hear the stomach's "I'm full" signal.

Please note, it takes roughly twenty minutes for the stomach to tell the brain it's had enough. Your stomach not only has no teeth, it doesn't have a voice. The only voice it has is one of gas, bloating, and irritability.

How many of these simple principles do you have in your lifestyle? Does your lifestyle need an overhaul? Can you afford to make some simple adjustments to get out of harm's way?

Time for PIES

Physically, have you been dealt some genetic "cards" you need to deal with?

You may want to undergo a DNA buccal swab test, which can tell you about your health, metabolism, and exercise profile. This exam may be the secret to saving your physical health.

Known information is easier to handle than unknown information. Personally, we think everyone should undergo this test.

Intellectually, has your family history led you to resignation about your health?

Do you need to evaluate your mindset around health and disease? Are you just accepting that you may get cancer because it's part of your family history? Are you being proactive in areas of prevention?

Take action on your intellect. Answer the above questions as they relate to your life. Are you setting yourself up for cancer when you don't have to? Do you need to take some action steps instead of being resigned?

Learn, learn, and learn some more. Without adequate information, it's increasingly difficult to make quality decisions. If the risk factors are there (outside of the normal behaviors we've discussed), find out and take action.

Emotionally, have you been living in an environment of toxic thoughts and emotions? What will you do to change this and care for yourself?

Evaluate all your relationships. Do they feed you? Do they harm you? Are you spending your time investing in the wrong areas? Are there areas in your life that need forgiveness? Are there people you need to connect with?

Allow us to share a personal story. Recently I (Mark) observed an encounter that dramatically impacted my life. The scene, between my wife and her mother, took place in a retirement home near Dallas, Texas. As I describe this event, please remember this: say what you need to say, because one day you may not be able to say it.

Dr. Michele and I walked into a room where her mother lay. Her mother has suffered for over fifteen years with debilitating conditions, both physically and mentally. I can't imagine being in that position myself and often wondered about the thoughts of this woman as she lay there unable to walk.

Each time we went to visit, the topic of conversation was basically the same. Do you know who this is? How are you? I love you. The visits were obviously always a highlight, even though they may not have been remembered for long. I reassured my wife that these visits, as difficult as they might be, were well worth the effort.

We routinely ended each visit in prayer, thanking God for the opportunity of the moment and asking for His peace in the situation.

This particular visit, however, was different. There had been much weight loss since the last time. There was a different feel in the air. The conversation began in the typical way but quickly changed tone after only a few minutes.

I watched my wife begin to tear up as she held her mother. Her mother became very lucid, and the conversation at once seemed very clear between the two. There were words of thankfulness and gratitude as well as looks of mutual love and respect. I sat motionless observing this moment. My wife's sweet mother, unwavering in her faith, seemed to be saying goodbye in her special way.

For me, this moment caused a pause in time. I thought to myself how many times I had failed to recognize moments like this in my own life. As the meeting drew to a close, the customary prayer was offered. I held my visibly shaken wife's hand as we exited the building down the long hallway.

My wife looked at me and said, "I know this is the last time I will see my mom alive. I can see it in her eyes." What a powerful statement!

Just a few days later, sweet Sara left this planet and changed addresses to eternally reside in the kingdom of Heaven. Say what you need to say. Never take for granted the moments or the people. Every moment deserves your greatest and best attention, because they'll never repeat themselves.

I offer this story in honor of my wife, Dr. Michele, and her mother, Sara. Additionally, however, I offer it to all of you. Let go of toxic emotions because they can eat you alive—literally.

One additional resource we can offer is Dr. Don Colbert's book, *Deadly Emotions*. It's a great read on this topic.

Spiritually, do you believe your choices can make a huge difference in your health? Cancer is a disease of the mind, body, and spirit. A proactive and positive spirit will help the person with cancer become a warrior and survivor.

Anger, unforgiveness, and bitterness put the body into a stressful and acidic environment. Learn to have a loving and forgiving spirit. Learn to relax and enjoy life. Life is a miracle that's meant to be enjoyed, not simply preserved.

We understand that cancer can be a frightening disease. However, it does not mean it will.

8

High Blood Pressure

WHAT IS HIGH BLOOD PRESSURE, ANYWAY?

From a medical perspective, we'll illustrate high blood pressure or hypertension with this example. Imagine you're holding a rubber band between two hands. Stretch it out just a few inches, putting a little tension on the band, then release it by bringing your hands closer together. Now, repeat the gentle stretch and release.

Our lives are meant to have a little bit of healthy stretch and a corresponding bit of relaxation. This keeps us, and rubber bands, elastic and balanced. But if you give it too much tension by stretching the band too far and holding it in a stretched state for too long, it won't spring back to its original shape and size.

If you stretch a rubber band too far, it snaps. The same is true with our physiology, intellect, emotions, and spiritual life. Too much tension might not immediately break us, but it's damaging nonetheless. We'll lose the ability to bounce back, and this carries cardiovascular risk, as well as the risk for emotional dysfunction, spiritual bankruptcy, and other physical diseases.

Hypertension

Hypertension (high tension) is another name for high blood pressure. This tension is located in the vessel walls of your cardiovascular system. Let's call it your internal vascular highway system.

As with other diseases, there's sometimes a genetic predisposition to hypertension, and our families also pass along to us unhealthy eating and living habits. We add to this tension by saying yes to everything and no to ourselves, which can spin our lives out of control.

The ACE gene codes for the angiotensin-converting enzyme is part of the renin-angiotensin system, which controls blood pressure by regulating the volume of fluids in the body. Studies show that patients with essential hypertension (high blood pressure) have two copies of a particular insertion allele, the II on the ACE gene. Those with this particular insertion allele have a significantly higher blood pressure with increased high salt intake and poor nutrition compared to wild type (normal) genes.

Incidence of hypertension was found to be significantly lower among individuals who reduced their sodium intake and improved the rest of their nutritional lifestyle. Yes, nutrition does affect how our genes act. We have more control than we think.

The standard American diet is hypertensive by its very nature. Unhealthy foods stress the body, causing high tension in our systems, which are trying to cope. And food isn't the only way we stretch ourselves. Most people suffering from high blood pressure are violating all the laws of our natural rhythm, from the time we get up to the time we go to bed.

Circadian Rhythm

Circadian rhythms are physical, mental, and behavioral changes that follow a roughly twenty-four-hour cycle. They respond primarily to light and darkness in your environment.

Light is the main cue influencing circadian rhythms, turning on or turning off cells that control an organism's internal clock. The hypervigilance with which many people live life has a big effect on the rhythm. Most tend to burn the candle at both ends.

Circadian rhythms can influence sleep-wake cycles, hormone release, body temperature, and other important bodily functions. They've been linked to various sleep disorders, such as insomnia. Insomnia will drive stress hormone production and in turn increase internal tension.

Abnormal circadian rhythms have also been associated with obesity, diabetes, depression, bipolar disorder, and seasonal affective disorder.

Our biological clocks drive our circadian rhythms. The biological clocks that control circadian rhythms are groups of interacting molecules in cells throughout the body. A "master clock" in the brain coordinates all the body clocks so they are in synch with each other.

The "master clock" that controls circadian rhythms consists of a group of nerve cells in the brain called the suprachiasmatic nucleus, or SCN. The SCN contains about twenty thousand nerve cells and is located in the hypothalamus, an area of the brain just above where the optic nerves from the eyes cross.

Are your eyes getting crossed yet with all these medical terms? Don't worry, there's no test at the end of this book. We simply want to be thorough and ensure that you have enough information.

A poor lifestyle will disrupt and aggravate the biological clock, interfere with its rhythm, and make it difficult to find health and balance unless these factors are addressed.

How are we destroying our natural circadian rhythm? We rise several hours before the sun comes up in the morning; we go to bed far after the sun sets and the moon comes up at night. By doing this, we set ourselves up to fight against our body's natural internal clocks, which are designed to follow the rhythms of nature.

By pushing the system with artificial lighting, jolting alarm clocks, electronic gadgets, and stress, we're disrupting the HPATG axis—hypothalamic, pituitary, adrenal, thyroid, gonadal— and creating a state of high tension. Our newfound hypervigilant state puts us at risk for hypertension.

In order to keep up with our high tension state, we stimulate with caffeine, amphetamine pills, sugars, energy drinks, and whatever it takes to achieve bursts of energy.

Are we suggesting going to sleep at dusk and rising with the sun? Since this is the way we're designed, that would be the recommendation in a perfect world. With the high demands of today's work world, we have to find a way to obey the laws of nature and still meet the demands of modern life.

The point is to cooperate as much as possible with the natural stretch and release we're designed to live in.

The circadian rhythm is designed to respond to the work and rest cycles of day and night. Our entire beings need this, including digestive enzymes, cortisol, adrenaline, testosterone, and other functions. When we disrupt the circadian rhythm, we're disrupting the natural processes in our body. Everything from the way we think, to the way we breathe, to the way we digest, and to the way we release tension in our four-part being is tied into these rhythms.

There are some very helpful medications that can help people move out of dangerous levels of hypertension. But in nearly all cases, this should be a stepping stone—in consultation with your doctor—to deal with all sources of tension in your life.

Every medicine has side effects. Every action has consequences. If your doctor scribbles a prescription without asking about the other tensions in your lifestyle, you're not receiving the best, most compassionate and helpful, care.

Am I Hypertense?

Did you skip the previous paragraphs and jump here? That might be an indication.

But seriously, do you always drive your car like you're delivering an organ for transplant? Do you talk fast, work fast, and multitask fast?

These stresses are toxic to the system and will cause high tension. Do you get stressed just *thinking* about sitting down and resting? Listen, it can happen to anyone. Just stay with us, and we'll teach you a better way.

In America, so many people are addicted to busy. Because of this, they can't really rest, because they've forgotten how to rest.

Here's a test to see if you're hypertense, or have hypertensive tendencies. Put your cell phone in another room, put your pets in another room or outside, turn off the TV, and sit in silence for fifteen minutes.

If the very *thought* of this experiment makes you stressed, you have the tendency to be hypertensive. If you can do this, but really want to grab your phone or go to your computer, you have the tendency to be hypertensive.

If you can't make it for fifteen minutes, you get an A+ in hypertension.

Fear and Other Stressors

Hyperstress is "normal" in our society. And, as you're learning in this book, "normal" is a terrible standard by which to measure our health and lifestyle.

We see people all the time who are emotionally drained—not living, just existing. There are physiological consequences of stress. In fact, high blood pressure is often driven by fear: fear of not making enough money, fear of not living up to expectations, and, ironically, fear of disease. You don't have to live like this.

We're both pretty high-energy people, so we've had to address stress and tension in our own lives. For me (Michele), medical school was a great example of how to build insane amounts of tension on the way to burnout: one-hundred-plus-hour work weeks, on call 24/7, in the Intensive Care Unit for seventy-two hours straight when on call. And the cycle continues week after week. It was a training ground on how *not* to live. Yet this is the way medical professionals are being trained.

In recent years, medical schools have finally come to the realization this lifestyle isn't good for residents. But an eighty-hour work week is still normal—and still unhealthy. This is one example of how the circadian rhythm gets out of balance.

Almost every physician or clinician is, in my opinion, stressed and depressed when they graduate medical school. They all don't ask for antidepressants, but many are hooked on caffeine and unhealthy food. And these are the people we rely on to help bring total-being wellness into our lives.

Modern medicine has made wonderful advances through the years, especially in the past century. But the trend has also been to separate physical health from emotional health—and intellectual health and spiritual health. This compartmentalization is a problem, because it ignores the reality of our design.

We have to visit these principles every day. We force ourselves to have a vacation about once a quarter. And when we get away, we disconnect. On our most recent trip, it took us about three days to really unplug and feel like ourselves again. That's why we recommend three-day windows of time to de-stress.

We also set aside one night per week as a date night, where we'll go to dinner and sometimes watch a movie. Why do we go to a movie? We want to give our minds a chance to go somewhere else, but we're very careful about what we watch.

If we don't purposely make an intentional effort to take breaks, we won't. Modern society is all about busyness. It's not easy to take a break (remember the fifteen minutes of quiet experiment?), but it's possible.

And if you want to improve your overall well-being, reducing stress will actually help you get in shape and maintain your progress.

How to Get in Shape and Stay in Shape

A common statement we hear in the clinic is, "I've lost the same forty pounds—for years."

Losing weight is the number one resolution made by Americans. Over a third of the population wishes to "exercise" and "stay fit." It's easy enough to start an exercise and diet program, but the trick is to find what gives you steady results over the long run.

With proper education and lifestyle management, you don't have to be a victim of chronic sickness and disease. Here are six tools for staying in shape.

1. Know your body composition. This means to know your body fat percentage and lean mass percentage and to keep them in the appropriate range for optimal health and well-being.

   We use body composition as a vital sign in the clinic. Remember, normal body fat percentages for men range from 10 to 20 percent and 18 to 28 percent for women.

   Ditch the scales. We advise against using just scale weight. Composition gives you a measure of muscle. We all want to maintain muscle mass. Muscle mass gets us around and keeps us active in the activities we enjoy.

2. Say no to sugar and fat with confidence. We often say yes to sugary treats and fatty meals in order to not hurt someone's feelings. There's a way to avoid toxic, inflammatory, foods

politely. And if someone gets upset about your choices, they don't have your best interests at heart.

It's been said that food is medicine. When it's *not* medicine in the form of fresh and raw fruits, vegetables, good clean meat, fresh and raw nuts and seeds, it can be poison. Realize that everything you put in your mouth matters. What we eat has an effect. It may take years to show up, but it will show up, with either health or illness. It's your choice.

3. Never overeat. Your stomach is the size of your fist. If you keep this in mind and stick to this rule, you'll do yourself a big favor. Your stomach doesn't have any teeth, nor does it have a voice.

4. Get smaller dishes. We recommend using eight-inch diameter plates and putting the larger plates away. This ensures that you stick to the concept of not overeating. Focus on serving sizes. With your new smaller dishes, help yourself to only one serving.

5. Think long term. We often think and feel invincible. However, things change. Treat your body with respect. Your heart has a lifespan of beats. Conditioning your heart is important in keeping it strong, but to push it beyond measure may shorten its lifespan. Thinking long term with your daily health decisions will help your body stay healthy longer.

6. Exercise in moderation. We all know exercise is important for long-term health of your heart and bones. We also know exercise maintains lean mass and helps control fat mass. It may be of great benefit to have your genetic profile tested to see exactly what type of exercise your body best responds to. Use this in order to set the right exercise routine. Remember, your body reacts positively to the healthy tension of exercise.

Staying in shape is the best way to ensure a high quality of life. We hear too many folks say, "If I had only known I'd live this long, I would've taken better care of myself." Don't let these be your words. Instead, have a vision for health, and make it a reality every day.

You were designed to live with a balance of healthy stress and rest.

Time for PIES

Physically, take at least fifteen minutes to sit in quiet.

Perform a body scan from the tip of your toes to the top of your head. Check in with your body systems. Do you carry tension in one area more than another? How long does it take for your body to be completely tension free? How is your breathing cycle? Is it short and shallow? Long and relaxed?

This is a key time to "own it" if you're hypervigilant. Don't miss this incredible chance to be honest and take the first step in learning to chill out.

Intellectually, remember it might feel like unhealthy food helps your state of mind, but it's actually stressing your whole being. Instead of heading for the ice cream, have a glass of water and go for your favorite walk.

Challenge the urge to relieve stress with food by adding a squeeze of lemon or lime to your water or listening to rejuvenating music on a walk.

Are you up for the challenge? How about taking a fifteen-minute walk right now? Many studies validate the idea that walking can metabolize adrenaline and help the body relax. Side note: we're all given legs to move, so let's quit making excuses and get after it.

Emotionally, come to terms with stressors like fear and anger. Sometimes it's not what you eat but what eats you. What's eating at your insides that makes you tense? Identify your greatest fear right now. Go ahead. Think about it. When it comes up, just say it. Once you do that, the emotional healing can begin, as well as the rational thinking to address the issue.

Spiritually, have you decided on an accountability partner for your journey? It's critical to find someone to be your buddy. Don't try to do it alone. Find someone to help you. Take some time with this. Interview a few people. There must be trust and authenticity. Remember, tough love is oftentimes the most promising. You know the saying, "Faithful are the wounds from a friend."

To bring down tension, and increase your enjoyment of life, be passionate about rest and fight to disconnect from stressors. It's worth it.

9

The Disease of Depression

THE INTERNATIONAL CLASSIFICATION OF DISEASES RECOG-
nizes depression as a disease. And so do we. What is depression?
It's the apathetic, blue, fatigued, tired, mood stemming from an
array of sources. Whether you're emotionally struggling, spiritually struggling, financially struggling, or physically struggling,
depression is a symptom. And it's a state of mind.

There are FDA-approved drugs available to treat depression.
In the professional medical community, depression is considered
a "mental disorder." That's one of many reasons why patients are
reluctant to say, "I'm depressed." They're afraid they'll be put
on medication. They're even more afraid of being classified as
mentally ill.

There are times when people have a chemical imbalance
or a diagnosis of post-traumatic stress disorder (PTSD). Other
times, hardships and tragedy can cause depression. Ups and
downs are part of life. We all go through hard times. But we
weren't designed to stay down.

We aren't immune to negative feelings, either. We sometimes
go into states of grief over disappointment because of our desire
to see people live well.

When one part of your four-faceted being isn't well, every other part suffers too. When you have a cold, your emotions and intellect are affected. When your mind and feelings are out of sorts, your spiritual life often suffers.

Disappointment can affect us on all levels as well. In fact, the Bible says, "Hope deferred makes the heart sick" (Proverbs 13:12).

We don't want to discount the fact that there is true clinical depression. There are some people who are born with the inability to make serotonin or dopamine. Their brains just don't make the amounts they need to be physiologically happy. That's where the clinician comes in and takes the time to understand the person physically, intellectually, emotionally, and spiritually.

Most people don't fall into this category. But few understand the interrelated causes of depression which we have control over.

Gut Feelings

Believe it or not, food can affect your mood. Brain function and emotions can be helped—or hurt—by the foods we eat or don't eat. After all, our brains are physical organs and rely on physical nutrients. A higher level of negative gut bacteria can drive toxic neurotransmitters like glutamate, glycine, and chemicals, which become irritants to the brain. The role of the gut microbiome in depression is a new discovery that is largely driven from the standard American diet. Bacteria become populated in an unhealthy way and secrete their byproducts into the gut. Usually these are eliminated, but in the case of small bowel bacterial overgrowth (SIBO), these byproducts can be reabsorbed and become neurotoxic.

Serotonin, with its precursor 5-hydroxytryptophan (5-HTP), is a monoamine neurotransmitter. Biochemically derived from tryptophan, serotonin is primarily found in the gastrointestinal tract (GI tract), blood platelets, and the central nervous system

(CNS) of animals, including humans. It's popularly thought to be a contributor to feelings of well-being and happiness.

Approximately 90 percent of the human body's total serotonin is located in the enterochromaffin cells (specialized cells) in your gut. This is a powerful link in the brain-gut connection. Unhealthy eating can disrupt the health of these special cells and decrease their ability to produce this happy neurotransmitter. When these cells become unhealthy, mood declines, appetite increases, and sleep becomes unpredictable. We begin to suffer in body and in mind. Cognitive functions, including memory and learning, decline. Does this sound depressing? Sounds like the perfect time to seek comfort.

For those who turn to food for comfort, this can become a downward spiral. Feel bad? Eat junk. Eat junk? Feel bad. Time for medication—the effects of food don't work. Many antidepressant medications cause weight gain. And weight gain can make a person more depressed. Unfortunately, this vicious cycle is common for many people.

The longer you live the standard American lifestyle, which drives sickness and disease in the gut, inflammation gets higher and higher. This can cause serotonin to get lower and lower— and all four facets of someone's being can spin out of control.

Many medications are classified as serotonin reuptake inhibitors or SSRIs for short. These drugs don't make more serotonin, they just allow your body to use what it already has in a better way. In other words, there is no such things as a deficiency of that class of drugs. So the drug is not improving the function of gut health, where 90 percent of serotonin is produced, and the drugs aren't giving it the precursors and nutrients to make more. It's just a band-aid to help you to use what you already have in a better way. Coming off these medications becomes very difficult because the cells that make serotonin still aren't working efficiently.

This is not to say that medication is all bad, but how about improving foundational health and using less medication? How about improving foundational health and weaning off medication? How about improving foundational health before we destroy health in the first place?

Walking Mummies

Those in the medical community who over-prescribe medications without addressing root causes have created a situation where people are walking around covered in band-aids.

That's what the world largely sees as healthy or acceptable. "I have my seven prescriptions to manage my sicknesses." But in reality, that person is sick. And dying. Is management really what we want to do as health care providers? No. Most of us entered medical school with a heart and passion to cure chronic sickness and disease.

We had a male patient who tried eight different antidepressants, and none of them worked. He said he was ready to try something new. What he didn't want was another pill and another side effect to cause another ill. We said, "Please just give us ninety days, and let's go on an anti-inflammatory nutrition protocol and see what happens."

In that ninety days, he wasn't completely healed, but he said he didn't hurt like he used too and had a little more energy. From there, we had him start exercising and eating less inflammatory food. We also put him on a probiotic to repopulate the good gut bacteria.

He came in three months later and told us, "Well, I cut my antidepressant in half." (This was done in consultation with his primary care doctor, of course.) We were moving in a healthy direction.

We began to fill in the functional foundation and put him on some 5-HTP and some melatonin at night, along with some magnesium. We also started filling in his nutrient deficiencies and driving serotonin production.

Three months later he had lost thirty pounds and felt much better. And yes, he stopped taking medication for depression. Today, he's on no medication and has lost over forty-five pounds.

Do you know the real key in this success story? It was him finally saying, "I'm ready for change. I've tried all these drugs and they aren't helping."

Chronic depression is like being stuck in a self-imposed prison—and not knowing how to get out.

Unlocking Freedom

So what are the steps to freedom from depression?

If you're waiting for us to say, "Test, don't guess," congratulations!

Self-medication and guesswork are dangerous. Consult with a trusted professional.

You must know some specific information about what's happening with your neurotransmitters, which involves what's called a neurotransmitter test to measure glycine, glutamate, serotonin, dopamine, epinephrine, norepinephrine, and more. This helps assess the chemical balance in your brain.

One recommendation we suggest, with the agreement of your doctor, is changing your nutrition to improve the microbiome in your gut. If you don't change this, you're not going to produce the right chemicals, in the right quantities, for a healthy brain. The voice of the bowel remains irritable. Does IBS (irritable bowel syndrome) sound familiar? Wouldn't you be irritable if you were constantly being bombarded with poor nutrition? We personally don't blame the bowel for getting "irritable."

First, we need to stop eating certain inflammatory foods and replace them with anti-inflammatory foods. We call this an anti-inflammatory nutritional protocol. If 85 percent of the immune system surrounds your gut and 90 percent of serotonin is made in the gut, this sounds like a good place to start first. Healing your gut, by putting the right nutrients in every day, moves you rapidly in the direction of a joy-filled life. Sounds like the perfect antidepressant to us.

The anti-inflammatory nutritional protocol means eliminating sugars, grains, processed foods, MSG, soy, high-fructose corn syrup, and other toxic foods. Some people must eliminate more if they have allergies, which are confirmed after being tested. You have to eliminate what's coming in and causing harm so that the body can heal and start to detoxify.

We add fresh and raw fruits and vegetables, clean proteins (hormone and antibiotic free), nuts, seeds, and plenty of fluids. Give the body what it needs and it begins the natural process of detoxification and healing. When we feel better, the body can begin to detoxify from negative emotions and moods like depression.

Second, a simple outside walking program is usually a positive addition. Air can be three times more polluted inside than outside. The body needs fresh air. That's one reason why people have such glorious times on vacation. Experiencing the wonder and beauty of the outdoors is a great way to combat depression and enjoy peace. Taking a walk outside in the sunshine is healing to the mind, body, and soul.

Positive activity metabolizes adrenaline (the stress hormone), and that's something we need to practice every day to manage stress.

Omega-3 Fatty Acids

More than 90 percent of the patients we test with an omega index are deficient in omega-3 fatty acids.

Omega-3 fatty acids are important for normal metabolism.[11] We're unable to synthesize omega-3 fatty acids, but we can obtain the shorter-chain omega-3 fatty acid ALA (alpha linolenic acid) through diet and use it to form the more important long-chain omega-3 fatty acids, EPA (eicosapentaenoic acid), and then from EPA, the most crucial, DHA (docosahexaenoic acid).

EPA and DHA are omega-3 fatty acids your body doesn't make, so we need to make these a part of our dietary intake. Your brain is more than 60 percent fatty acid material. So if some were to call you a *fathead*, you may as well say, "Thank you." Please understand, proper levels of good EPA and DHA in your brain is like changing the oil in the engine of your car. Your mind will run more smoothly and last longer with the right nutrients.

There is evidence that omega-3 fatty acids are related to mental health, including that they may tentatively be useful for the treatment of depression. There's a link between omega-3 and depressive mood. The link between omega-3 and depression has been attributed to the fact that many of the products of the omega-3 synthesis pathway play key roles in regulating inflammation, such as prostaglandin E3, which has been linked to depression.

Many Americans have been misinformed about fats, thanks to the nonstop messaging about "fat free" foods. In the process, most people are fat-deprived. Sounds strange, doesn't it? Women need to supplement three grams of omega-3 fatty acids and men need about four grams per day.

There are good omega-3 fatty acids and bad omega-3 fatty acids. We ask patients about the supplements they take, and almost every time they show us a bottle of omega-3 pills from some big-box store. Check the label. Many supplements tout 1000 milligrams, but when you read the label you'll see each dose contains 60 milligrams of EPA and 40 milligrams of DHA (a total of 100 milligrams of the good stuff) and 900 grams of other omega-3. Ninety percent of the pill has no potency.

It's not fish oil you need, it's omega-3 essential fatty acids— EPA and DHA. Fish oil can be a source of these nutrients, but it's not the fish oil we need. We've even seen fish oils marketed as gummies. These usually have trace amounts of EPA and DHA and large amounts of sugar. And we now know sugar is poison and can actually feed depression and mood swings. The first time we saw "gummy" fish oils for kids, we nearly fell over. Who in their right mind would invent this garbage for kids?

Quality Sources of EPA and DHA

The most widely available dietary source of EPA and DHA is oily fish, such as salmon, herring, mackerel, anchovies, menhaden, and sardines. Oils from these fish have a profile of around seven times as much omega-3 as omega-6. Other oily fish, such as tuna, also contain omega-3 in somewhat lesser amounts.

Krill oil is a source of the omega-3 fatty acids, EPA and DHA.

Omega eggs produced by hens fed a diet of greens and insects contain higher levels of omega-3 fatty acids than those produced by chickens fed corn or soybeans. In addition to feeding chickens insects and greens, fish oils may be added to their diets to increase the omega-3 fatty acid concentrations in eggs.

The addition of flax and canola seeds to the diets of chickens, both good sources of alpha-linolenic acid, increases the omega-3 content of the eggs, predominantly DHA.

Flaxseed (or linseed) and its oil are perhaps the most widely available plant source of the omega-3 fatty acid ALA. Flaxseed oil consists of approximately 55 percent ALA, which makes it six times richer than most fish oils in omega-3 fatty acids. A portion of this is converted by the body to EPA and DHA, though the actual converted percentage may differ between men and women.

Omega-3 fatty acids are formed in the cells that make chlorophyll of green leaves and algae. While seaweeds and algae are the source of omega-3 fatty acids present in fish, grass is the source of omega-3 fatty acids present in grass-fed animals.

Reasons to Be Positive

You have many reasons to be positive about your future. The main reason we want to highlight is that when it comes to depression, so many positive changes are within your control and within your reach today.

A little bit of investment today will affect your tomorrow. The key is consistency.

Just like a little baby begins by rolling over and then moves onto his or her hands and knees, the consistent effort is what makes progress possible. When babies keep trying, they'll eventually stand up and hold themselves up against the couch; then they'll take their first step. Before you know it, two years have gone by and now they're running around.

That's the way your process has to be. Determined and stubborn in failure. We encourage you to be ruthless and relentless in your pursuit of a positive mindset.

No parent gives up on their child when they stumble and crawl; so why do we give up on ourselves?

Why can't we believe we will run too? Why don't we believe we'll enjoy health to age eighty and beyond?

It's possible.

Time for PIES

Physically, remember that physical movement positively affects your whole being. And enjoyable movement, like taking a walk or exercise, improves your outlook and self-esteem even more. When you move, your body improves the neurotransmitters that help make your mood, and attitude, happy.

Intellectually, you now know how nutrition impacts your brain. We hope this fact gives you hope. If you suffer from depression or simply feel down more often than you'd like, there are steps you can take to help your whole body improve. The simple ninety-day elimination plan is a place to start. Stop putting in what could be contributing to pulling you down.

Emotionally, remind yourself there may be external factors affecting your feelings. But you are not powerless. Changing the foods you eat and adding enjoyable exercise are within your control. This may be the time to address the situations, people, and places that drive you to comfort foods. List these areas and begin deleting the power they have over your life as you replace the kneejerk reactions of reaching for food for comfort with something that will provide you the health and vitality you desire.

Spiritually, pause and see the bigger picture of the road ahead. You didn't arrive where you are in one day. And it will take many days to fully realize your goals. But if you take daily steps, you'll get there—and enjoy the journey.

10

Autoimmune Diseases

THERE'S A LOT WE DON'T KNOW ABOUT AUTOIMMUNE DISEASES. But there's much we're learning, and can bring to the battle.

In basic terms, "autoimmunity" means eating itself. The body begins to eat itself or fight against itself.

At present there is no clearly defined cause-and-effect relationship for many ailments called "autoimmune disease," such as Parkinson's, Lou Gherig's, multiple sclerosis, muscular dystrophy, and ailments including arthritis and allergies.

What we do know is that autoimmune diseases are on the rise in our nation. The more research on the foods and beverages we consume and the way they're broken down in the gut, the more links we're finding to these diseases.

Leaky Gut

A common link to many of these autoimmune diseases appears to be "leaky gut syndrome." At present, this condition is known to exist, but researchers are unsure about what causes it or exactly what to do about it.

Those who suffer from leaky gut routinely complain of bloating, gas, abdominal cramps, food sensitivities, and various aches and pains that can't be pinpointed. It's a condition that appears to be marked by a failure of the lining of the small intestine, which allows substances to leak into the bloodstream in an abnormal way. People who've been diagnosed with celiac disease and Crohn's disease often experience this occurrence.

Researchers are also linking a person's diet and their chronic stress level to leaky gut syndrome. While these two factors may not directly lead to leaky gut, medical practitioners do report that patients with ailments associated with leaky gut do experience significant relief of their symptoms if they follow a prescribed nutritional plan and simultaneously reduce their stress levels.

We've seen many autoimmune conditions improve or even disappear once an anti-inflammatory food protocol is employed. I know we harp on this a lot, but removal of sugars, artificial sweeteners, MSG, fried food, soda, processed foods, and refined grains are the key to getting this "leaky gut" condition under control and seeing relief from autoimmunity.

There's also interesting research on "excitotoxins"—chemicals that impact brain function. The culprits appear to be preservatives, food additives, genetic modifications to foods, and various food processing procedures. Again and again, researchers advise that a person avoid all MSG, all hydrolyzed proteins, and hydrogenated fats.

How can you know if the foods you're eating have these substances? Check the labels on processed foods before you buy, including both packaged and canned goods. Become informed about the many ways these additive and filler substances are being "defined"—there are unscrupulous processors and manufacturers who are using "new words" for old additives. (We frequently blog and send email newsletters about new medical discoveries. Subscribe to our email newsletter for updates.)

Another syndrome that may be linked to both leaky gut and autoimmune disease is irritable bowel syndrome. IBS, as it's often called, has many of the same symptoms as "leaky gut," with the notable addition of diarrhea or constipation. Exact symptoms vary widely. Some studies have linked hormonal changes and the use of antibiotics to IBS, in addition to foods and stress levels.

Emotions and Immunity

Someone who's living in an emotionally toxic lifestyle situation may develop an autoimmune disease against a certain glandular tissue because of their unhealthy emotions.

We can't point to a particular study, but the medical community agrees stress does affect our physiology. In our experience, there's a correlation between toxic emotions, toxic behaviors, and autoimmune symptoms. We also see poor nutrition as a root of autoimmune disease, and this seems to confirm the leaky-gut theory.

A large percent of our immune system lines our gut. It's located in the mucosa- associated lymphatic tissue (MALT), and gut-associated lymphatic tissue (GALT) that's right under the microvilli, the finger-like projections that line the intestinal tract. Microvilli are microscopic cellular membrane protrusions that increase the surface area of gut/intestine cells and are involved in a wide variety of functions, including absorption, secretion, and nutrient transport. Thousands of microvilli form a structure called the brush border that's found on the surface of the small intestines that line the gut lumen. We realize these are fifty-cent words, but hang on, we're trying to give you a general understanding of how this can all go right or go wrong.

Microvilli function as the primary surface of nutrient absorption in the gastrointestinal tract. Because of this vital function, the microvillar membrane is packed with enzymes that aid in the breakdown of complex nutrients into simpler compounds that are more easily absorbed. For example, enzymes that digest carbohydrates called glycosidases are present at high concentrations on the surface of enterocyte (intestinal cell) microvilli. Thus, microvilli not only increase the cellular surface area for absorption, they also increase the number of digestive enzymes that can be present on the cell surface.

Nutrition affects the inner lining of the gut, which is made up of this brush border of microvilli. As we barrage the microvilli and the enterocytes with the standard American diet, the cellular glue that holds these microvilli together can begin to break down. This is analogous with bombs being dropped on a large flat plain. After repeated impacts, damage to the once-smooth surface is permanently achieved. Obviously, this is a vast oversimplification, but you get the idea. When gaps open up, high molecular proteins or food products can get past the lining.

The first line of defense in the GI tract (intestine) is the gut microbiome, the healthy intestinal flora that should normally inhabit your gut. The second line of defense is the microvilli/ brush border. The third line of defense is the MALT and GALT, neatly organized into an immune system called the Peyer's patches of the gut.

Because the lumen (passageway) of the gastrointestinal tract is exposed to the external environment, much of it is populated with potentially pathogenic (harmful) microorganisms. Peyer's patches thus establish their importance in the immune surveillance of the intestinal lumen and in facilitating the generation of the immune response within the mucosa. If the first and second line of defense begin to fail, these Peyer's patches are placed on high alert. The immune system now starts reacting to foreign invaders, and autoimmune disease is on the horizon.

Basically what can happen is the passageway becomes damaged, which is caused by the constant presence of poor food choices, and dangerous substances are allowed to pass through, alerting the body that foreign invaders and unnatural substances are present.

We're designed to be healthy, but if we use the analogy of a car, you can't put bad fuel into a car and expect it to run well.

The lining of the gut is very resilient, but eventually it breaks down if it's continually exposed to a poor diet, chronic stress, and overuse of antibiotics and medications. This lining of strength and resilience breaks down. It becomes permeable or leaky. A leaky gut is born. The medical literature refers to this as intestinal permeability, which is a real condition. Leaky gut and intestinal permeability are the same. This gut lining becomes leaky, and now large proteins are leaking in and the immune systems become activated. The Peyer's patches begin to protect the body by creating antibodies to these large molecular proteins that look very similar to cellular proteins—thyroid, kidney lining, bone, liver, and other cells. More autoimmune disease is born, worsening numbers of lupus nephritis, autoimmune hepatitis, autoimmune pancreatic disease, autoimmune adrenal disease, hashimoto's thyroid disease—all of these proteins are coming in, and the body is making antibodies to them that are very similar to tissue proteins, so you begin to make antibodies and destroy yourself.

Stop Fighting Yourself

Harmful antibodies often decline when a system is reformed by a change in lifestyle. When we stop ingesting the offending agents, the lining of the gut can begin to heal.

For our patients, after receiving a thorough exam, we recommend an anti-inflammatory protocol (yes, there's that term again), which usually consists of lots of plants, very little meat, and more fish. Probiotics also help heal the gut micro-biome, the first line of defense.

Every region in the gastrointestinal (GI) tract has a certain ecology that should exist there. Stomach PH is different from the small intestine's PH, for example. And each area in your gut has a different microbiome, with trillions of bacteria. Each of these biospheres is responsible for digestion; production of certain minerals, vitamins, and enzymes; breaking down food; absorption of nutrients; and immune defense.

Often, after a complete workup, the first step is to heal the gut with friendly bacteria. If you're thinking of *yogurt* as the probiotic you need, that's not the entire answer. Typical yogurt found in big-box stores only contains one strain of probiotic and often contains loads of sugar. Instead, look for a nonprocessed Greek yogurt in full-fat form.

The most important part of keeping the bacteria healthy is feeding them right with the nutrients they like to eat. Fiber is food for the friendly bugs in the gut. Get your twenty-eight to thirty grams of fiber every day without fail; it's vital to long-term health.

Fiber is considered a *prebiotic*. Prebiotics are typically nondigestible fiber compounds that pass undigested through the upper part of the gastrointestinal tract and stimulate the growth or activity of advantageous bacteria that colonize the large bowel by acting as substrate for them.

Other dietary fibers also fit the definition of prebiotics, such as resistant starch, pectin, beta-glucans, and xylooligosaccharides. A 2016 review stated that prebiotics are "food ingredients that help support growth of probiotic bacteria" or "nondigestible substances that act as food for the gut microbiota." Essentially, prebiotics stimulate growth or activity of certain healthy bacteria that live in your body.

If you have a sick gut, you may need to use a probiotic. Probiotics are defined as live microorganisms that are believed to provide health benefits when consumed. The term probiotic is currently used to name ingested microorganisms associated with benefits for humans and animals. These probiotics aid in reestablishing and maintaining intestinal health and digestive function. We often add probiotics for broad base repopulation and ongoing regeneration of gut bacteria for a period of time that is individualized for the patient.

The gut also calls for other nutrients of health, like glutamine. Glutamine provides cells in the digestive tract with a vital source of energy that's required for regulating their production and improving their efficiency and rate of nutrient absorption. Its role in strengthening the gut lining is well known. Glutamine also helps water absorption in the gut, aiding in hydrating the whole body—certainly a necessary component for good health.

By eliminating the incoming irritants and improving the first line of defense (the microbiome) with a probiotic, autoimmune disease incidence and aggravation decreases. Good nutrition and added nutrient support improve the second line of defense, the microvilli. The third line of defense is calmed down when the system is in balance and the environment is peaceful.

Who would've known that autoimmune disease can begin and end in the gut?

Proactive

While there's no singular remedy for autoimmune disease, irritable bowel syndrome, or leaky gut syndrome, much research points to three areas worthy of consideration:

1. Monitor Your Own Gut Function. These diseases and conditions can involve, to some extent, the digestive tract—especially the small intestine and large intestine. The health of these organs of the body—which are the largest organs of the body apart from a person's skin, measured in square inches—is often overlooked.

   People tend to ignore diarrhea and constipation, thinking these conditions are "normal." They are not. Pay attention to your gut. Listen to what it is telling you. And seek help sooner rather than later.

2. Consume Sufficient Fiber. Fiber refers to the "roughage" that remains after healthful nutrients have been digested and

absorbed from fruits, vegetables, and whole grains. Fiber can be consumed in a number of ways—it's even available in capsule form. An adult should consume at least thirty-eight grams of fiber a day for men under the age of fifty and twenty-five grams for women under the age of fifty. Though this number is generalized, please understand that some folks need much more.

Food labels now list dietary fiber among the ingredients on the package. Fiber has been shown to help lower cholesterol, prevent constipation, and improve digestion.

3. Consume Sufficient Water. The best "beverage" is pure water. By pure, we mean water without any flavorings or "juice" products added to it. One of the best investments you can make in your health is a water purification system. While the water in your city water system may be labeled "safe to drink," that label doesn't mean the water is pure—without harmful chemicals and "acceptable" levels of bacteria in some cases.

How can you know if you're taking in enough water? Take your current body weight and divide it by two. Then divide that number by eight (the number of ounces in a small drinking cup). For example, a person who weighs 160 pounds will calculate that half of that weight is 80, and that number divided by 8 will produce a result of ten 8-ounce cups of water a day. The number should be based on your ideal weight. We say "ideal weight" because a three-hundred-pound person (whose ideal weight is two hundred) doesn't need to consume 150 ounces of water a day. Obviously, activity and heat can increase the need for hydration.

That may seem like a lot, but few people drink out of containers that hold only eight ounces. If you exercise vigorously or perspire a great deal in your work, you'll want to consume even more water. Water "flushes" out your system, helps maintain cell health, and helps fiber function normally in your digestive tract.

We certainly don't claim that the consumption of fiber and water can prevent or cure autoimmune diseases, leaky gut, or IBS, but we do know this: in our wellness clinic we find that people who consume sufficient fiber and pure water do much better at regaining and maintaining their physical health than those who don't.

Time for PIES

Physically, take time to listen to your body. It's designed to tell your intellect how it's feeling and how it reacts to certain foods and activities. Don't ignore your body screaming at you through the voice of your gut. Listen, then make necessary adjustments to bring calm.

Intellectually, as we recommended above, realize that your body is talking to you. What is it telling you? Sometimes we all walk through life in a hurry, literally numb to the happenings around us. We need to re-educate our minds to receive and perceive information correctly. "What is happening in the here and now?" is a very important question that should be asked (and answered) often.

Emotionally, are you tired of allowing toxic relationships and stressful thoughts to dominate your life? Can you take steps to reduces these poisons? Your body will thank you. Good old fashioned pruning is performed to make trees or plants grow better. The dead branches are cut off and the energy of the tree is free to move further into generating life. No more energy wasted on dead branches. We must do the same in our own lives with emotions and relationships. Learn to set and enforce boundaries. This will make your life "grow" to its fullest potential.

Spiritually, you want the best for your loved ones. You want them to be healthy in every area of their lives and to make good choices about their whole being. Do you love yourself the same way? Learning to love yourself is so key. Being honest and true to yourself is the first step. Do you care about yourself? Really? We are serious. We all have the right to be honest in this answer. If you don't care about yourself, please acknowledge it . . . and know that you will by the time you finish this book. Friend, loving yourself is critical. We want you to experience true health in all areas of your life as well as true love for yourself. When you love yourself, you can truly love others. Without self-love, selfless love is impossible.

11

Food for Thought on Alzheimer's and Dementia

NOT ALL DEMENTIA IS ALZHEIMER'S DISEASE, BUT ALL dementia is disconcerting to those who experience it. These brain disorders can be devastating to caregivers also. It's emotionally, physically, and often financially exhausting.

Dementia by definition is a broad category of brain diseases that cause a long-term and gradual decrease in the ability to think and remember. The decline is so great that it affects a person's daily functioning. Other common symptoms include emotional problems, problems with language, and a decrease in motivation. A dementia diagnosis requires a change from a person's usual mental functioning with a greater decline than one would expect due to normal aging.

Vascular dementia refers to the type of reduced mental function which occurs after a stroke. The vascular system is our network of blood vessels that supply blood through the body. This type of dementia is often reversible, as is dementia related to thyroid function and certain vitamin deficiencies, as well as dementia due to blood pressure abnormalities. However, if vascular dementia goes unchecked, its consequence can become a permanent loss of the ability to think and live an independent life.

Alzheimer's disease, also referred to simply as Alzheimer's, is a chronic brain disease that usually starts slowly and worsens over time. This type of dementia is what we're most familiar with. It's the cause of 60 to 70 percent of cases of dementia. The most common early symptom is difficulty in remembering recent events (short-term memory loss). As the disease advances, symptoms can include problems with language, disorientation (including easily getting lost), mood swings, loss of motivation, not managing self-care, and behavioral issues. As a person's condition declines, they often withdraw from family and society. Gradually, these individuals experience even long-term memory loss, and bodily functions decline and cease to operate optimally, which can ultimately lead to death. Although the speed of progression can vary, the average life expectancy following diagnosis is three to nine years.

The cause of Alzheimer's disease is poorly understood. About 70 percent of the risk is believed to be genetic, with many genes usually involved.

One example is APOE genotype, a gene linked to vascular disease and dementia. The APOE gene can be accelerated with toxic living, or inflammation. Driving the inflammatory cascades faster and harder with an inflammatory lifestyle can cause Alzheimer's and vascular dementia to show up earlier and earlier. Just because one has the genetic predisposition doesn't mean a person has to develop Alzheimer's disease. In other words, if the genes say "likely," you have the power to make them say "unlikely." We encourage everyone to take action to drive the genes down to the unlikely highway.

Other risk factors include a history of head injuries, depression, or hypertension. The disease process is associated with plaques and tangles in the brain. A probable diagnosis is based on the history of the illness and cognitive testing with medical imaging and blood tests to rule out other possible causes. Initial symptoms are often mistaken for normal aging. Examination of brain tissue is needed for a definite diagnosis.

That's the trouble with receiving an accurate diagnosis of Alzheimer's disease—the condition can only be fully diagnosed during an autopsy. Although that's a bit late for a remedy, there are steps we can take to reduce risks.

If you suspect dementia/Alzheimer's disease in yourself or a loved one, consult a physician sooner rather than later. There are many ways to help slow the decline of brain function, and in some cases, underlying biological causes can be eliminated to great benefit.

We all fear losing our minds. It's refreshing to know we do have some control over our long-term outcome. If we choose regular physical exercise, avoid eating inflammatory foods, and avoid obesity, we may decrease the risk of Alzheimer's and other types of dementia. As we have said in previous chapters, our bodies are intimately connected. From the food we eat to the thoughts we think, we have more control over our long-term outcome. Let's instill hope as we look at putting out the fire. We can relate brain dysfunction/dementias to a fire in the brain. This fire is chronic inflammation.

Putting Out the Fire

In most communities, the fire department has personnel and trucks stationed to put out fires. Our inflammation system is designed to put out fires too. Without inflammation, we would die. For example, if you get a thorn stuck in your arm, what happens? Inflammation comes to the rescue to surround the wound, encapsulate it, swell up, and push it out.

After the fire department puts out the fire, they go back to the station house, rest, and wait for the next call. That's acute inflammation. It occurs on an as-needed basis.

Further described, acute inflammation occurs when you have a wound, such as skinning your knee. The affected area forms a scab, swells, and goes into healing mode. The immune system comes to aid and protect you from hurting the area again. The scab, the redness, the heat—the inflammation—is a protective measure for the short term of less than three months.

Systemic or chronic inflammation is like a fire department receiving an emergency call and then receiving many more calls. While they try to put out one fire, they have to send limited crews all over to fight the other fires.

Before long, there are fires all around town. The firefighters are exhausted, spread too thin, not getting any rest, and becoming ineffective. That's exactly what happens throughout one's system with chronic inflammation.

When inflammation becomes chronic, the immune system and the immune cells are overreacting and creating inflammatory mediators every day on an ongoing basis. And those inflammatory mediators include: NF-Kappa B, IL 6, tumor necrosis factor alpha, and more, which are at the root of mind/body disease that results from inflammation. These signals are cellular mediators that the immune system spills out into the system, in effect saying, "Hey, there is a war going on here!"

This inflammation causes vascular damage and harms the nervous system, potentially increasing the progression of Alzheimer's disease and other types of dementia. In some people, inflammation causes vascular disease and it shows up as heart dysfunction—congestive heart failure, atrial fibrillation, high blood pressure and hardening of the arteries, whereas in other people inflammation shows up as vascular disease that affects the brain and contributes to the development of vascular dementia.

Ever heard of a transient ischemic attack (TIA)? These mini strokes can contribute to the development of dementia.

Of course we see some natural progressive changes with an aging brain, but diseases of the brain are unnecessarily increased with unhealthy lifestyle and chronic inflammation.

It's a vicious cycle and a domino effect all rolled into one.

Since we're now well aware that all chronic sickness and disease starts with inflammation, it stands to reason to focus on keeping the fire of inflammation at a minimum. This is the way to keep disease at bay. We can't overemphasize how the body sees and reacts to everything we ingest. The persistent pollutant load from the standard American diet, all of the stress we're under, and the environments we reside in, all affect our systems in particular ways. The immune system goes from hyperalert and overactive to depressed and exhausted.

Poor diet causes the immune system of the gut to overreact, which creates inflammation in the vascular system, contributing to diseases of the heart, kidney, liver, and brain. This is a systemic response. We see patients with all kinds of diseases, but the root cause is often inflammation brought on by the standard American diet and poor lifestyle choices—agitating the immune system every day.

Brain Food

Life is in the blood. That's a biblical principle. The blood carries vitamins, minerals, nutrients, hormones, and everything our brains need to function.

You wouldn't feed your dog or cat garbage and expect it to be healthy. So why would we expect our blood and brain to thrive on junk food?

The most important medical decision you make every day is at the end of your fork. With every bite, think, *Is this harmful or helpful? Is it medicine or poison?* Yes, that's right, food (or *un-food*, as we like to call it) can be poison.

Good food for the brain also consists of positive thoughts, affirming emotions, peaceful media input, encouraging conversations, and plenty of rest.

Remedies and Tips

Not *every* person suffers from dementia or brain disease as they age, although you may think some do because of the goofy things they do. Obviously, we are just injecting a bit of humor here as we talk about this very serious matter. Listen, folks, there are people well into their nineties who score very high on tests related to brain function. Let's be one of those people. Here are four areas any person can include in their lifestyle to improve general brain health:

1. Continue to Learn. Challenge your brain daily with new information and stay curious about your world. We recommend reading nonfiction books. Challenge your brain with problem-solving activities such as crossword puzzles, Sudoku puzzles, anagrams, and memory exercises. Memorizing something every day helps keep the mind in top form. Consider learning a new language or learning even more about health. (Great job reading this book, by the way!)

2. Whole-Brain Activities. Engage in activities that tap into both sides of your brain. If you play a musical instrument, practice daily. If you don't play an instrument, you may want to learn how. (Simply listening to music is good, but it is still passive.) Conversations challenge a person's intellect and emotions. Find someone you enjoy conversing with and talk!

3. Eliminate All Brain Toxins from Your Diet. Eliminate all MSG and other substances called "excitotoxins." These substances overstimulate neuron receptors. The neuron receptors allow brain cells to communicate with each other, but when they're

exposed to excitotoxins, they fire impulses at such a rapid rate that the neuron receptors become exhausted. Three of the foremost excitotoxins are glutamate, aspartate, and cysteine. Your body needs a degree of glutamate, but not in the form of monosodium glutamate (MSG), which is added to many foods. Aspartate is related to some artificial sweeteners. It's a highly problematic substance that is best avoided whenever possible. Cysteine is a fairly common food additive known for artificially creating "flavor." High levels of cysteine have been correlated with Parkinson's and Alzheimer's disease.

4. Spend Daily Time in Prayer or Meditation. As part of your quiet time with God (or even your understanding of Him), give voice to areas for which you are thankful. An attitude of gratitude should be voiced out loud. This may sound like a very simple approach to preventing or helping with dementia issues . . . but consider the fact that the person who voices thanks is calling upon memory function and speech generation. Expressions of gratitude are also enhanced by writing them down. Journaling is a wonderful way to engage both sides of the brain as well as your spirit. We'll use a well-known saying here: "Your attitude determines your altitude." Let's all learn to have high-altitude brain function.

The Gift of the Present

The topic of Alzheimer's and dementia reminds us of the wonderful gift we can enjoy today: the present moment. Take care of your body, and your body will take care of your mind. Use your days to make a wonderful lifetime of memories you can enjoy for many more years. Make sure you experience the blessing of now before it becomes a distant memory. This simple awareness will make memories much sweeter.

Time for PIES

Physically, are you feeding your brain the right food for thought? We all know that garbage in yields garbage out. Let's put great thoughts in right now. Say the following phrases out loud, where your brain can clearly hear:

- I am successful.
- I am happy.
- I am joyful.
- I love life.
- Life loves me.

Yes, there are many more, as well as variations. Please expand and use these habitually.

Intellectually, are you exercising your brain like a "muscle"? Never think you've learned all you're designed to learn. There's always something new. If you think you have it all figured out, you're in danger of becoming cynical. Cynicism, in turn, can drive us to downright negativity. Make a decision to adopt a new hobby or goal. Make sure it's challenging. In this challenge, you'll find brain power.

Emotionally, are you afraid of diminished mental function as you age? Channel that energy into resolve, to care for your entire being. Never let fear become your driving force in life. Fear can take you places you never need to go and make you do things you never wanted to do. Being mentally sharp requires effort. Let's put the effort into areas that give us passion and reason for living.

Spiritually, engage your thoughts on words of hope and peace. Probably the saddest situation is someone that's lost hope. Hope keeps us going. We trust this book gives you hope and inspires you to become what we desire to become—hope dealers to our family, friends, community, and the world.

12

Working with a Wellness Professional

YOU MAY CONSIDER MOVING FORWARD WITHOUT THE HELP OF a professional, but why would you do that? We all have a doctor or clinician we rely on for medical ailments, so why not choose one that has wellness rooted in how they practice?

Perhaps you've had a bad experience with a doctor, clinician, or coach, but that's really no excuse. In fact, we wrote this chapter to help you search and find one of the many wellness professionals who can work with you—and help you avoid those who won't be a good fit.

Ethics and Responsibility

In simple terms, medical ethics boil down to this: do no harm and give the patient autonomy. It's really about partnership in wellness.

Essentially, a medical professional should deliver the best information and insights, but the decisions should be yours. And the first decision you must make is what kind of care you want: *sick care* or *well care*.

If you're looking for a *sick care professional* to treat symptoms with a smile and a "pill for every ill," we can't help you. (And neither will *sick* care professionals.) Frankly, a doctor who prescribes pills without also prescribing changes in lifestyle is unethical. Why? Because they took an oath to do no harm, and they should be giving their patients every option to experience health.

But if you're looking for solutions to health challenges and are willing to make changes (not just take pills), you can experience *well care*. You want to work with a doctor/clinician who puts the responsibility back on your choices and helps you make the necessary changes. After all, you live with yourself 365 days of the year. Who does most of the responsibility lie with? The answer is, "the person looking back at you when you look in the mirror."

In other words, you don't want to fall prey to the ICI *(I caused it)* syndrome if you have the potential to choose a better way. There is no such thing as guilt when it comes to lifestyle, only consequences. What one who wants long-term quality health desires is not to fall into the pitfall of accepting the last half of life being riddled with chronic sickness and disease. Who wants to take a pill for every ill when we can do something about it? You want to choose the right practitioner.

The practitioner can be the guide, but you must take the right steps. We can lead a horse to water, but we can't make him drink. The path to wellness isn't always easy. Choose your hard. It's hard to be obese, diabetic, hypertensive, and have to take ten pills every day. It's hard to prepare your meals, eat right, and stay in shape. Choose your hard. The right practitioner will engage with you and help you reach your wellness goals. Their heart is as invested in your health as yours.

A wellness professional aims to keep your human engine performing in top condition, always. They'll point out where you're running into a health crisis before the crisis occurs. This allows the opportunity to completely avoid a negative and life-destroying event. They're invested in helping you maintain your body composition, maximize your biomarkers and keep them in the normal range, as well as keep your fitness levels optimal to meet your personal needs.

Questions and Challenges

When we first meet a patient, we'll ask questions like, *What's this visit really about?* and *How prepared are you for change?*

Then we'll go a little bit deeper and ask, *Just how ready are you to get rid of that bowl of ice cream everyday? What's your capacity to grab onto the opportunity to be completely and totally well, physically, intellectually, emotionally and spiritually?*

We're looking for raw, honest answers. The state of readiness determines success. If one isn't ready, change won't occur. If mindset is right, change is eminent in an upward direction. That's the basis for a positive, transformative, doctor-patient relationship.

You must take an active, not a passive, approach to your relationship with your doctor. Remember, we are all patients to a doctor somewhere. We all need to honestly answer the question, "Do I really want to get well?" If the answer is yes, the question becomes, "How badly do I really want it?"

And ask your own questions as well. If the practitioner doesn't perform an in-depth evaluation of your biomarkers, body composition, and fitness capacity, we'd suggest finding another practitioner. Remember, your medical professional works for you.

You Might Need a New Doctor If . . .

With apologies to Jeff Foxworthy and his "You might be a redneck" routine, here are some signs you may need to change doctors.

If your practitioner has a can of diet soda sitting on his or her desk and tells you not to drink diet soda, that might be a good time to say, "Thank you for your time" and leave.

If you've been going to a certain doctor for ten years and he or she has never asked about your consistent weight gain, you might need a new doctor.

If your conversations usually include your favorite brands of cigarettes and whiskey, it could be a sign you need a different doctor.

If your doctor weighs more than you and your spouse put together, maybe it's time to shop around.

If your doctor thinks biomarkers are pens used to draw tattoos, you might want to ask for a new referral.

If you and your doctor are drinking buddies, you might need to find a new doctor. (Of course, you can still be friends.)

You get the idea. Your health is serious business, and you need a committed partner to be successful. Choose wisely.

A Word to Our Fellow Professionals

All kidding aside, we really love and respect all doctors and wellness professionals. It's a tough career, and the pressure can be overwhelming. Patients don't always want to get well.

Many of our patients have been medical professionals, and we want to help you succeed personally and professionally. There's a better way to help patients, but it's a road less traveled.

We realize it's tough to change course. Many of us were taught to follow an algorithm of ordering tests, diagnosing, and prescribing a drug. Based on the outcomes we see in our society, more and more doctors are looking for better ways to practice too.

We hope this book is helpful, and we'd be honored to meet you. We want you to be able to thrive and lead by example. Shouldn't this be a driving motivation for being a wellness practitioner? Lead by example. How can we teach others to be completely well if our personal lives don't demonstrate this foundation?

Weight Loss Programs

If you've found a cheesecake that's as healthy and nutritious as a tree-ripened pineapple, please send us the recipe. If you've found a lasagna that lowers your cholesterol, bring a pan over to our office.

Otherwise, please don't waste your time and money with so-called "medical weight loss" programs, especially those that focus on drug use to lose weight and never address permanent lifestyle change. This is absolutely a joke in regard to betterment of health and should be avoided.

The standalone goal of "weight loss" is a band-aid at best and deceptive at worst. Remember, we've seen many "skinny diabetics." How many times have you seen people try and fail at weight loss plans and end up worse than they started? The goal must be less excess fat and more muscle, or the plan is doomed to failure before it starts.

The Bloated Leading the Bloated?

We had a patient we'd been working with for a very long time, trying to get his nutrition and lifestyle turned around. We finally asked, "What is your primary care physician doing? Where does he stand in all of this?"

He responded, "Well, when I share about my desire to be more fit, he doesn't really listen to me. He writes my prescriptions and sends me on my way." This patient saw him for medication management and saw us for wellness.

We often get the opportunity to speak at medical conferences. We'll often ask by a show of hands how many doctors in the audience know their body composition or the status of their inflammatory biomarkers. We're always astonished, as the number of hands raised is usually less than 10 percent. Our point is, to be successful, you need a team united around the same vision for wellness.

The doctors attending our session understood our message and began to change their nutritional lifestyle. The overwhelming calls and response to our medical office regarding their appreciation and how they'd made changes in their practices was truly remarkable. You can't change what you don't know. We often get stuck in a rut and don't even know there's a better way.

The previously mentioned patient's physician was one of the medical doctors attending one of the conferences at which we spoke. Several months later, when our patient had his next appointment, he was stunned. His doctor had lost forty pounds. "Wow, doc, what happened with you?"

The doctor responded, "I finally decided to listen and gave up the yellows and the whites." (The *yellows and whites* refer to sugar, grains, and breads.) "I'm going to lead by example."

As our patient shared this story with us, he added, "Now I'm more apt to listen to that doctor." And he did. Together, they encouraged each other on their journey, and their results are having a ripple effect throughout their families and community. They have a relationship built on trust.

Find a practitioner who will listen, who will invest in himself or herself as well as you, who won't let you settle for "normal," and who will try to find the root causes for your conditions.

Benefits of Finding the Right Wellness Professional

In addition to helping you address the consequences associated with the negative FRAUD emotions (as discussed in an earlier chapter), the right wellness professional can help you in the following areas.

- **Develop a Can-Do Attitude.** Attitude is a huge factor in what a person will decide to do—from filling and taking a prescription, to following a wellness plan, to addressing the emotional and spiritual issues that may be holding back their progress.

Attitude also directly impacts how quickly a person will get well from an existing ailment and how the person will persevere in developing new wellness habits.

We're always a little surprised when we recommend a change and find the patient quickly reacting with a firm, "I can't do that. I just *can't.*"

We don't give up. Instead we inquire, "Who told you that you can't?"

I (Michele) recall one person looking at me as if to say, *What does that have to do with anything?* I continued, "Somebody *taught* you that you are incapable of doing what I suggested. You weren't born believing that. I'm curious to know who taught you that you can't."

Henry Ford is quoted as saying, "If you think you can or think you can't, you are right." We believe Ford was right!

- **Confront Your Excuses.** Beyond saying "I can't," a person may be prone to justifying his or her acknowledged bad habits—those statements of justification can take a wide variety of forms with a high degree of certainty. A good wellness professional will confront your excuses for what they are: *excuses.*

  Excuses are rampant in our world. Below are a few we hear rather frequently in our clinic. We've even provided an excuse-busting truth for each one. (You're welcome!)

  Excuse: I don't have time to go to the gym.

  The Truth: Everyone on this planet gets paid the same amount of time per day: 1440 minutes. *How* you spend the time you're given is your choice.

  Excuse: I don't feel like it.

  The Truth: You don't feel like it because you're not doing it. The more you don't do it, the more you won't feel like it.

Excuse: I don't want to give up my sweets.

The Truth: No one requires you to totally give them up. We simply tell you about the poisonous ingredients. When you believe the truth, your *want to* will change.

Excuse: I don't have support at home.

The Truth: Unfortunately, many times we see patients in our clinic who have little support from their family. If this is true for you, we understand your pain. Find a wellness professional who can support your journey. In time, your example will make an impact on those around you.

Excuse: I won't have any fun if I make all these changes.

The Truth: You sure won't have any fun while you're lying in bed, chronically sick, taking numerous medications, and experiencing regret. Being healthy increases your ability to get the most out of life.

Excuse: I guess I just have a chemical imbalance.

The Truth: Some people do have chemical imbalances. However, most chemical imbalances are disguised by, and sometimes caused by, emotional excuses.

Excuse: I'm just too stressed. You just don't understand what I have to deal with.

The Truth: If you think you have no power to make a positive response, you won't even try. One of the best ways to combat stress is through action.

Excuse: I just feel like giving up all the time.

The Truth: Every person has feelings of being overwhelmed at times. There are plenty of people around you who would encourage you, if you'd ask.

Excuse: I don't want to explore my spiritual life, I've been hurt by the church.

The Truth: So was Jesus, at least by the religious leaders of His day. When you start feeling sorry for yourself, remember Him. Furthermore, people always hurt other people— sometimes intentionally and sometimes accidentally. That's why forgiveness is such a miracle, and such a necessity for healing.

Excuse: I don't need to see a doctor (or find a more suitable doctor). I'm not any more sick than my friends.

The Truth: "Normal," in today's America, is not healthy. Taking uncomfortable steps now will make all the difference in your life and in the lives of your loved ones.

Every successful athlete has a coach. For you to successfully improve your wellness in every area of life, you need the right medical professional. It truly is a life and death decision.

Time for PIES

Physically, have you made a complete assessment of the physical symptoms you want to speak with your doctor about? Now is the time. Be proactive and inquisitive. The end result is confidence in your wellness plan. If you're not sure of something, ask until you're satisfied.

Intellectually, and honestly, does your doctor take a proactive and preventative approach? Or does he or she prescribe a pill for every ill? It's hardcore introspection time. This is about your health, not loyalty. Your goal is prevention and healing, not reaction.

Emotionally, are you afraid of seeing a medical professional? Are you concerned about the possibility of changing doctors for fear of hurting feelings? As stated above, feelings can't matter in regard to wellness. What is best for you is best for you. It's that simple. *Do you really want to get well?* If the answer is yes, do what you have to do regardless of emotion.

Spiritually, are you building a reservoir of desire and determination for change? What can you do to develop this further? Does confidence burn inside you? How about hope? How about passion? These should be exploding right now in your heart of hearts. If not, snap out of it and realize how special and valuable you are to the world. Nobody else can be you. So be the best you that you can be. It's all about internal passion and hope. These are the prerequisites of confidence.

MOVING FORWARD TO WELLNESS

At this point in the book, we want you to know more about who we are, what makes us tick, where we come from, and what gives us our passion.

Mistakenly, some believe we were blessed with a "silver spoon" life or that wellness has come easily for us. But this couldn't be further from the truth. We've endured tragedy and hardship, which began almost at birth.

We were both given up for adoption and had pretty rough childhoods. We can both relate to the word *abandonment*. Our birth parents didn't have abandonment on their hearts but experienced terrible circumstances. Maybe that's why we're so committed to supporting each other and our patients. Often, there doesn't seem to be a way out. We both worked against all odds, one day at a time.

Michele's Story

As a young girl, I chopped wood, shoveled snow, raked leaves, and delivered newspapers to earn enough cash to buy things our family couldn't afford.

In high school, my grades were a disaster, probably because of the mix of stress and learning challenges from changing schools twice between first and twelfth grade. But I loved music, which is probably the reason I didn't drop out of high school. By ninth grade, I was composing music and played a total of eight instruments—some better than others. But I also loved sports, including track, volleyball, basketball, and especially martial arts.

After years of work, I reached black belt status in Tae Kwon Do and became a three-time state champion and was ranked tenth in the nation. Competing in the Olympics started to look like a real possibility.

One week before my second national tournament, I had a major injury to my left knee. What an injury it was—I tore every possible ligament. In one moment, my martial arts career was over. I felt hopeless.

Shortly thereafter, I found myself homeless and was forced to live in my car for close to eight months. I kept a loaded gun under my pillow since I was afraid of the dark. Of course I had friends, and I often found myself on their couches, downstairs in their basements, or in a spare bedroom.

When I finally could rent an apartment, I slept on the floor and used candles to save money on electricity. My goal was to rehabilitate my knee, but I couldn't afford a physical therapist. So I joined a gym.

It was there I learned to train with weights properly and discovered a new passion—bodybuilding.

In 2006, after winning five state competitions, I entered the national bodybuilding arena and won both the NPC USA and IFBB North America Championships heavyweight class. And in 2007, I won both the NPC Masters Nationals and NPC USA heavyweight class.

In the late 1990s, I decided to center another new arena: osteopathic medical college. Thanks to the generosity of a friend, who offered to pay for my first semester, I jumped in and never looked back. I chose to be osteopathic because osteopathic doctors had a philosophy and understanding of the four-part person.

I completed an internal medicine residency and a sports medicine fellowship. I hung a shingle and have moved progressively toward healing patients one at a time. My life of healing really accelerated when I met the love of my life and soul mate, "Dr. Mark."

The point, and our reason for sharing these stories, is to show we understand tough circumstances and can relate to intense emotional pain.

Most of all, if you knew how unlikely it was that I would ever be called "Dr. Michele," you'd be as amazed as I am.

Mark's Story

I shared earlier that, as a young teenager, I was clumsy and "husky." I was picked on and bullied, and those voices still try to echo in my mind.

I channeled my fear and pain into athletics, even though it didn't come naturally to me. Baseball became a passion of mine, and I played in college and went on to play professionally in Australia for one season, earning rookie of the year. I dug in and dug my way out, or in this circumstance, I climbed to the top.

After my career ended, I needed a job. So I decided to serve my community in a unique way—as a police officer. Mental and physical conditioning was crucial in my career as a police officer. I served ten years on the SWAT team, climbed the ladder to sergeant, and retired after twenty-four years.

During that time, I also fell in love with bodybuilding, traveled the world performing feats of strength with a Christian ministry, and met the love of my life, Michele. I am called to teach others how to be completely and totally well. I truly desire to help people find the missing piece that gives them total peace in their hearts and in their lives.

As you already know, my mother's suicide impacted me greatly. In a weird way, instead of discouragement, it gave me more courage to never stop encouraging people.

After police retirement and returning to my studies, I became a naturopathic doctor. Believe me, there aren't many people who would've thought I could become "Dr. Mark." On top of it all, I now get to work with the queen of my heart daily, in the process of healing people's minds, hearts, and bodies.

The point is, you never know how your journey to wellness might positively impact your life, career, and relationships.

We both understand how life can deal some harsh blows. We know the world will lie to us about who we really are. Turning the other cheek is scriptural, and when the card is dealt, one has the opportunity to see what's truly rooted in the heart. We love the challenges.

Moving away from our past can seem as impossible as un-ringing a bell. We've both had times when we wanted to give up. But it's possible, and amazing, to reinvent your life and become the person you were meant to be. Each and every day, Dr. Michele and I do just that. The awesome part is, we get to do this together.

Moving Forward

So far in this book you've explored a lot about yourself, about the diseases many people dread, and about making a decision to not settle for "normal."

Most of all, we want you to grasp how much hope there is for your health and your life.

As we go through the following chapters, take time to actually implement what you're learning, in all four facets of your being. This way, you'll benefit from our encouragement as we move forward together.

Let's get started!

13

Setting Goals and Making Plans

We've all heard about, and perhaps experienced, the negative side-effects of financial debt. But do you have "wellness debt"?

Over time, you may have neglected physical wellness: exercise and eating correctly. You've "talked it" but not actually "walked it." Excuses become routine. Fatigue begins to increase, along with the numbers on the bathroom scale. As a result, your ability to handle life's stressors decreases. You find yourself feeling on edge more often than not.

On the outside, you glare at yourself in the mirror and realize the person staring back at you doesn't look as healthy or vibrant as you'd like. You might think, *I really need to start exercising.* Or you might even declare, "I'm going to start working out next week." But next week never arrives.

Just like financial debt, wellness debt didn't accumulate overnight, or even in a month. In the same way, you should realize you'll need patient, sustained changes to improve your wellness.

When setting goals and making plans, you'll need to simultaneously give yourself a break and be lovingly honest with yourself. Give yourself a break and recognize that short-term "fixes" won't work. So don't try another crash diet or an unrealistic exercise plan. Be lovingly honest with yourself by not being brutal. Don't beat yourself up, but face the facts. You're worth investing in!

Facing the Facts

We ask patients the question, "Do you believe the foods you normally eat are good for you?" The answer is usually no.

Then we continue, "Okay, we both agree. Do you love yourself? And do you love your family?" And the answer, at least to the second question, is a confident yes.

"Do you give your children ice cream?"

"No," they exclaim.

"But you just said it wasn't good for you. Why would you want to hurt yourself and your family, even a little bit?"

At that point, people either make the connection or try to steer the conversation toward the nearest exit. People know what is inherently good or bad for them. What most don't understand is why they intentionally sabotage their health.

We all need to come face to face with the truth. When you face the truth you have an opportunity to make a decision. It's an opportunity to choose freedom.

So the person with an emotional attachment to certain foods—in this example, ice cream—must ask himself or herself, "What would it be like to *not* want ice cream? Can I imagine that? What would it be like to *not* comfort myself with food?"

Do you love yourself enough to stop hurting yourself?

Start Simply to Failure-Proof Your Goals

You have to failure-proof your goals, especially as you begin. In society, and maybe in your experience, failure is almost expected.

For example, when we're trying to change the food we eat, we may set a goal to eat one serving of fresh vegetables every day. That's not hard. Or an early goal might be to bring two bottles of water to my desk every day and drink them instead of sugary drinks. Simple.

The point is to develop a habit of forward progress and minimize setbacks. Even in the examples above, the amount of joy and satisfaction you'll experience with "small" successes will surprise you.

We've told patients, "In thirty days you'll be in a different place, your blood pressure will drop and start to normalize, your excess fatty tissues will begin to drop, and you'll be using new, smaller loops in your belt."

One goal we often suggest to women is, select an outfit they want to wear and hang it in the closet where they can see it. When they are too small for their current wardrobe, they can give their clothes away and make someone's day. By the way, if you keep clothes that are too big, you're subconsciously setting yourself up to fail. We want you to set yourself up to win!

Your Really, Really, Real, Real Reasons for Wellness

You may want to lose weight, feel better, and enjoy exercise. But we all need our own deeper reasons for wanting to be well. And these reasons are connected to the life we want to live, the person we want to be, and the example we want to set.

God created you with a very specific purpose for this particular time on the earth. Understanding these three aspects of your being will help you set goals—and hit them!

#1: Your unique design

Every person is born with natural aptitudes and innate gifts. These have been present in you from birth. Many people find it helpful to go back in their memories and remember what they enjoyed doing most during age four to seven.

Even if your favorite activity was to build forts out of discarded Christmas trees or ride a bike or play dress-up, those play activities likely provide a window on what you truly *enjoyed* doing and on what you had no doubt about being "good at."

When you combine what you're good at with what you truly enjoy, you can live more intentionally in your purpose.

God gifted you for a reason. Enjoy rediscovering the many gifts God placed on you.

Take a moment to write down your understanding of your unique design and the gifts God has given you. Here are three examples from our patients:

- *From the time I was a little girl, I loved to teach my dolls and stuffed animals, to talk to other people about ideas, and to read and write. I grew up knowing that this is why God put me on this earth. At present, I am a teacher, and I write and publish fiction during my summer months away from the classroom.*
- *God gave me a logical mind, capable of dealing with principles, step-by-step procedures, and also good eye-hand coordination. I do well in things like woodworking and building. You guessed it, I work as a building contractor and a master carpenter. I specialize in building churches.*
- *I was never an indoor kid. I liked being outdoors, and by the time I was five years old, I had a "garden" growing in my mother's flower bed. Instead of a tricycle, I had a riding toy tractor. I knew by the time I was a teenager that I was going to be in some area of agribusiness the rest of my life . . . and I am. It is what fits me.*

If you're like most people, your current circumstances include a mix of areas you are gifted in and areas that drain you. Clearly defining those is a powerful first step in setting the right goals.

#2: Identify an Area of Service

Your highest purpose—and the path to a fulfilling, energizing life—is to serve others.

Ask yourself, *Who needs what I have to give?* Write down several people or groups of people you might help in practical ways in the next ninety days. This may be a person with health challenges, a neighbor who needs help around their house, or someone who needs a (healthy) meal.

#3: Establish Goals

Once you're on the path toward personal wellness, and on the path of purpose and service, it's time to set some goals and make some plans.

Identify two or more big goals you want to achieve in your lifetime. Focus on *who* you want to be as much as on what you want to *do*. Focus on your purpose and gifts, not on the material rewards or the compliments from others.

- Identify at least one goal (separate from your big life goals) in each area of your life: physical, intellectual, emotional, and spiritual. You must be specific.
- Create "sub-goals" for each of your major goals. These sub-goals are incremental and, in most cases, sequential. Think of them as "baby steps" toward your big goals.
- Put your goals on a timeline. For example, if your physical "big goal" is to lose twenty pounds, break this down into incremental goals of losing four to eight pounds per month for the next three months. This gives you a goal of losing about two pounds a week,

which is a good weight-loss pace that most people can maintain.

- Reward yourself for reaching incremental goals, but don't reward yourself with something unhealthy. In other words, don't reward yourself with a big slice of cake for losing two pounds. Equally important—don't beat yourself up emotionally if you fail to reach an incremental goal. Simply readjust your timeline and keep going.

Enjoy Setting and Reaching Your Goals

Recognize that it takes about ninety days for a habit to truly take root. Some say it only takes twenty or thirty days, but that's not realistic in our experience. It's generally much easier to "get back on the wagon" if you stay focused on a ninety-day goal.

Let's be honest. It isn't possible to stay at peak motivation all the time. Give yourself a break occasionally. Relax and enjoy the present moment. Spend time having pure fun with people you love. As many elementary school teachers know, students are often more interested in learning after they've calmed down from "recess" than they are ten minutes before a break.

Focus on total-being results. Change even one thing in your life for the better, and you'll reap total-being results. The more you tap into the goals that motivate you to develop self-discipline, the more your entire life will benefit. Wellness is a win-win-win-win proposition.

Tap into Brain Power

Your own brain is your greatest ally when it comes to making lasting changes in your life—whether it's related to physical health or to the other three areas of intellectual, emotional, and spiritual health.

Neuroplasticity is a new area of medical research. Generally speaking, neuroplasticity proposes that with each new brain experience (a thought, a stimulus, a perception, or an experience), the brain rewires itself slightly, and the end result is a restructured physical brain. This process takes time.

You've heard the saying "Practice makes perfect." The same is true here. Thinking practice makes thinking perfect. Your new thinking can become automatic and therefore the new normal.

The bottom line is that the brain allows us to learn to like new foods, develop new tastes, generate new ways of thinking, become more creative in certain areas of our behavior, and change our overall emotional orientation toward what is "good for me" rather than what only "feels good."

Exercise promotes the release of hormones in the brain called "nerve growth factor." These hormones are needed to keep our brains from *shrinking* as well as to keep areas of the brain well-connected. Our bodies and DNA were designed for movement. With less exercise, people lose strength, their muscles atrophy (shrink), and their joints become stiff. In addition, the brain doesn't receive the necessary hormones to stay healthy.

We know what you're thinking. *I know people who have forgotten to exercise their minds and have lost them.* Be nice now, friends. We all have room to grow.

The best way to keep both your body and your brain strong and well-connected is to exercise regularly.

Your Goal-Planning PIES

Here's a recap, and guide, for writing down your goals. And by the way, bringing these to your appointment with your wellness professional is a great way to begin the relationship and help you choose the right allies and accountability partners.

This is super important. People who fail to write down a vision don't really have vision.

The Foremost Gifts and Talents God Has Given Me

_____

_____

The Big Life-Goals I Desire to Achieve (Examples: Run a 5k race, take up a sport you used to love, hike up a mountain, take a family member on a trip.)

_____

_____

Who I Want to Serve
During the next ninety days::

_____

_____

In the next year or two:

_____

_____

Overall in my lifetime:

_____

_____

Specific Ninety-Day Physical Goal (Examples: Eliminate certain foods from your diet, walk five miles in one week, add a certain healthy food to your diet.)

_____

_____

Incremental Goals (Examples: Throw away one unhealthy food from your freezer or pantry today, buy a pair of walking shoes this week.)

_____

_____

Specific Ninety-Day Intellectual Goal (Examples: Become actively engaged in an activity that that utilizes a God-given talent, begin serving in an area that energizes you.)

_____

_____

Incremental Goals (Examples: Finish reading this book by next week, make an appointment with one wellness professional within the next three weeks.)

_____

_____

Specific Ninety-Day Emotional Goal (Examples: Make progress in FRAUDS—Fear, Resentment, Anger, Unforgiveness, Disappointment, and Shame.)

_____

_____

Incremental Goals (Examples: Study what the Bible has to say about FRAUDS tomorrow, forgive someone who has hurt you right now, seek forgiveness from someone you've hurt tomorrow, do something you want to do [but were afraid to] next week.)

_____

Specific Spiritual Goal (Examples: Assemble a team of accountability partners, evaluate if your current church [or lack of church] is meeting your spiritual needs.)

_____

_____

Incremental Goals (Examples: Ask one person to be your accountability partner this week, buy a book about a spiritual topic that interests you today.)

_____

_____

Use a calendar or planner to break down the big goals into smaller incremental goals. Map out a strategy and a plan for the next ninety days—and beyond.

14

Increase Energy and Health Symptoms

THERE ARE MANY TIRED PEOPLE IN THE WORLD, BUT RON AND Patti may have been the least energized couple ever to (slowly) walk into our clinic for an evaluation.

He was sixty-one and she was sixty years old. They'd been married almost forty years. Ron was a former athlete in high school and college, but he weighed almost 300 pounds. Patti was about 120 pounds overweight.

They had no energy and were drinking caffeine and consuming sugar all day just to keep moving. Even though they crashed at the end of the day, they slept poorly.

By now, you may be able to guess what we told them. "If you guys will trust us, adhere tightly to your personalized plan, and give it some time, you'll get results and feel so much better."

It is up to you to stay the course. You live with yourself twenty-four hours a day, 365 days a year. Only you can be authentic on your journey. We encourage you to stay the course and surround yourself with individuals who will encourage you on your path to wellness. We again stress this is not about a "diet," it is about a lifelong, whole-hearted lifestyle change.

When Patti and Ron started the process with us, they were taking blood pressure medications, cholesterol medications, anti-inflammatory medications, sleep medications, and pills for pain and joint dysfunction, and they were gulping down energy drinks by the six-pack. They had their own individual pharmacies, so to speak, making more trips to the pharmacy monthly than to the supermarket for groceries.

No wonder they were tired. In addition, their excess weight was draining energy from them twenty-four hours a day.

Every excess pound of fat tissue we carry is the equivalent of *ten* pounds pushing down on our joints. You have to account for gravity's powerful downward force. Would carrying a backpack full of rocks all day make you tired? That's what Ron and Patti were doing. When you think about it, some folks are carrying an extra "person" around all day long. Talk about having a monkey on your back!

After an initial round of testing, they began to work their plan. In thirty days, we saw significant results, and after nine months, Ron weighed 175 pounds, having dropped over one hundred pounds. Patti dropped sixty pounds. Because they focused on overall wellness and not some crash diet, they not only lost weight, their energy levels were off the charts—and the symptoms of unhealthiness either decreased or disappeared.

"I have more energy now than I did in college as an athlete, and I weigh the same as I did then!" Ron cheered.

As you begin to lose the excess fat, you will have more energy. By the way, Ron now has a six-pack for abs (not energy drinks in his front pockets), and his body fat percentage is what it was in his collegiate athlete days.

Prior to their program, Patti had been severely depressed. She walked with her head down and was ashamed of herself. Because they addressed all four facets of their being, they were also healthier intellectually, emotionally, and physically. And because they helped each other on the journey, their marriage relationship went from okay to great.

Now they both walk with their heads held high and attitudes toward life even higher. From fat, fatigued, and almost dead (as they put it) to fit, energized, and ready to conquer every day, they transformed their lives.

They're excited about the future. They aren't just living for the day anymore; they are living with energy and hope.

Don't Exercise

No, that's not a typo. We actually don't want you to dive into an exercise program until you're ready—and until you've established a relationship with a wellness professional.

You must understand that food is first. Your relationship to food trumps exercise. This does not mean quit exercising if you are already on an exercise program. This is for the individual who is getting started and has not had exercise as a regular part of his or her life. It is not uncommon for the body to go through a detoxification in the first three months and require more rest at first.

Exercise requires energy. If you don't feel good, emotionally or physically, do you think you'll stick with exercise? Be compassionate and understanding, begin listening to your body, and be realistic.

Begin with nutritional changes and include changes in your emotional and spiritual life. You will begin to feel better. As you do, and as your energy level picks up, start adding some enjoyable exercise to your day.

We will, however, strongly encourage everyone to move more and sit less. Getting a pedometer is ideal to count steps daily, with ten thousand being the goal. Energy cannot be made up; it must come from within. Exercise will eventually become more fun, stress relieving, and energizing.

Don't pretend you have energy—go get some real energy that will last.

Energy Drinks—The Good, Bad, and Concerning

We are often asked about energy drinks, so here's our take. So-called energy drinks are everywhere. Entire sections in convenience stores are dedicated to them. But are they healthy?

First, let's examine their active ingredient: caffeine. Caffeine has differing effects on the nervous, cardiovascular, and metabolic systems, depending on the quantity consumed. The average dose of caffeine (85–250 mg, the equivalent of three small cups of coffee) may result in feelings of alertness. Higher doses (250–500 mg) can result in restlessness, nervousness, and insomnia.

In high doses, caffeine can even cause hyperadrenergic syndrome, resulting in seizures and cardiovascular instability. A recent report, published by the FDA's Center for Food Safety and Applied Nutrition, cited sixteen deaths related to energy drinks. Yes, you read that right, sixteen!

Energy drinks contain substantially more caffeine than conventional cola or soda-type beverages. Many also contain caffeine-containing ingredients such as guarana and kola—or cola—nut.

Researchers once believed that the active ingredient of guarana was a chemical specific to the plant called guaranine. But they later discovered that it was just caffeine.

Kola nut, or cola nut, is likely safe for most people when consumed in foods in small amounts. In larger amounts, the caffeine in cola nut can cause insomnia, nervousness, nausea, and increased heart rate and respiration.

Adding these additional ingredients to an already highly concentrated caffeinated beverage can spike the caffeine levels substantially. The sugars and artificial sweeteners are also unhealthy. It is also important to know that caffeine is a toxin, for which the body must work very hard to expel. Sugars and artificial sweeteners, as we have discussed, are inflammatory, immunosuppressive, and even disease-causing.

Dependence on these type of energy drinks is detrimental to your physical health and possibly harmful to all areas of your being.

Symptom Relief

Sickness and disease bring symptoms of *dis-ease*. How does a person find relief from symptoms? There are two main ways.

First, there are drugs and physical therapies that help a person deal with severe pain, discomfort, depression, and biomarkers that are out of balance. We're thankful these are available, But they are not the best long-term strategy.

Second, the ultimate solution to relieving symptoms is getting to the root of the problem—and not just the physiological causes. Is there an emotional component? Are there relationship issues in play? Does the patient have a disease, or is her or she living an inflammatory lifestyle?

If an inflammatory lifestyle is at the root (and the vast majority of the time it is), we get on top of all those symptoms by decreasing all the inflammatory biomarkers through proper nutrition and lifestyle. And we deal with the other factors, including fear, resentment, anger, unforgiveness, disappointment, and shame (FRAUDS) that breed disease.

For example, depression (often left over from an emotional wound from a past event) often leads to weight gain, which leads to joint pain, which leads to inactivity, which leads to more weight gain, which leads to high blood pressure, which leads to heart disease and stroke. The root cause of all those physical symptoms and diseases is emotional depression. Yet many medical professionals treat the symptoms by prescribing pills for pain or high blood pressure.

What doctor do you know who digs into the root of depression before writing a prescription for an antidepressant?

Recently we "prescribed" to a patient, who happened to be a doctor, thirty minutes of silence while sitting in a chair, overlooking the ocean. He looked at us like we were nuts. However, after we explained the desired outcome in response to his symptoms, he understood. Guess what? When we saw him again, he told us that was the best medicine anyone had ever given him.

We must stop chasing symptoms and find the root causes of sickness and disease. When you do the work laid out in our plan, roots expose themselves and are allowed to resolve and heal.

Chasing the Vine

The worst long-term approach to symptom relief is selecting one symptom and prescribing a drug. All drugs have side effects, which create more negative symptoms. Sad to say, but this is part of the reason it's common to know someone taking ten or more medications at once.

Drugs are not bad. However, being irresponsible for your health, and failing to evaluate the FRAUDS in your life, is the tragedy we face in our health care system today. It is easy to take a pill for every ill, but it takes effort to solve the deep-rooted problems.

The good news is, once we get the roots out, not only do pills go away but so do the chronic diseases that wreak havoc on our lives.

Facing a symptom is like chasing a vine. If you just keep pruning the leaves, the vine will still grow. But if you start with the leaf and trace back to the branches and then onto the trunk of the vine, you'll find the root. Once you deal with the root, the vine will cease to grow and eventually die.

This is true of physical symptoms and also emotional and spiritual symptoms. For example, fear is a debilitating symptom and is often rooted in deeper issues of resentment, anger, unforgiveness, disappointment, and shame. Can you begin to see how responsible you are for the shape you're in? Let us help you find your way out.

Symptoms We Want

By moving away from the standard American lifestyle and eradicating inflammatory living—emotionally, physically, spiritually, and intellectually—biomarkers of health and body composition will improve. And now the symptoms can be positive.

We're all familiar with symptoms of disease, but have you ever considered the symptoms of wellness?

Symptoms of wellness can include joy, happiness, a sense of freedom, hope, motivation, increased energy, inspiration, feeling rested, and peace.

These are some symptoms of wellness. You can experience them!

Time for Pies

In each of the four areas below, write down the negative symptoms you are experiencing, along with the positive, healthy symptom you want to enjoy.

Physically, the negative symptom I want less of is _____.

And the symptom of wellness I want more of is _____.

Intellectually, the negative symptom I want less of is _____.

And the symptom of wellness I want more of is _____.

Emotionally, the negative symptom I want less of is _____.

And the symptom of wellness I want more of is _____.

Spiritually, the negative symptom I want less of is _____.

And the symptom of wellness I want more of is _____.

15

Less Fat and More Muscle

WHEN I (MARK) WAS GROWING UP, I WAS NOT ONE OF THE strong guys and certainly not one of the star athletes. I had good coordination and did pretty well in sports, but you wouldn't have known that from watching me walk down the street.

As an only child who didn't seem to fit in with any group, I got picked on. I even remember a big guy named Butch who thought it was funny to flick my ears as he walked by. He was baiting me of course, but what was I to do?

I spent a lot of time by myself but also remained very nice to everyone—even Butch. Frankly I was ashamed of who I was and ashamed of how I looked. When I was growing up, if you were chunky, even a little bit, you were fat. And that's how I saw myself. I didn't like my looks, hair, body, or even my thoughts about myself.

In high school, many of my teammates had defined muscles, six-pack abs, and big biceps. They could naturally run fast, jump high, and lift a lot of weight. Deep down, I was embarrassed that I wasn't as gifted.

I carried a deep sense of shame. But this experience now inspires me to try harder and never quit.

I ate anything I wanted—pizzas, sandwiches, and soft drinks. I remember eating half a loaf of bread every day. I didn't know any better. I was a bucket of inflammation before anybody knew what inflammation was. Food provided a comfort, but not the real comfort I was longing for.

In college, our baseball coach tried to keep an eye on our nutrition—a little bit. But I didn't really learn about wellness until I moved to Australia—on the other side of the world. Talk about a culture shock!

As a baseball player, I had nothing to do all until it was time to play ball each night. There was a gym down the street, and one day I decided to check it out. From that day on, I began to ask questions and apply myself to challenging exercise.

I started lifting weights and eating a little bit better. Guess what happened? My body started to respond. Little by little, fat decreased and muscle increased.

When I came back to my home town in the United States, I didn't know how much I'd changed, but my friends sure did. Yes, I had more muscle and less fat, but the overall experience increased my confidence and self esteem—little by little.

As a kid, being ten or twenty pounds overweight was "normal" for me. I guess that's why we are now so opposed to "normal" unhealthiness—because we remember how unhappy we felt, and how much shame that unhealthiness piled on our hearts.

We want you to know there is a better way to live. Even if you had a rough beginning, you can turn your life around. You don't have to be especially gifted—or muscular or athletic—to enjoy how you look and feel.

We know how tough it is to change your outward appearance, because it's so tied to your inward concept of yourself. Remember, your mind must lead the way; your body will follow.

Dropping the Heavy Armor

Fat is sometimes worn like a protective armor, shielding us from fear, resentment, anger, unforgiveness, disappointment, and shame.

People go back to the habits they learned as a child when they are under stress. It takes one time to learn something and a thousand times to un-learn it. You may be on a journey to wellness, but when you're stressed, your old habits will show their ugly heads every single time.

The healthier we get, the less time we spend destroying our lives with negative behavior. Once we know better, we are no longer willing to pay the consequences.

When we think about increasing muscle and decreasing fat, it's not just about *physical* muscle. We want you to be strong in your intellect, emotions, and heart too. We all need to grow and become stronger in those areas, because when you're strong, you can lift more and handle more resistance.

At the same time, we need excess fat to go away physically—and intellectually, emotionally, and spiritually. We must remove gluttonous behavior, insatiable thoughts, and lazy carelessness from our entire being and transform our whole lives. Materialism and consumerism are gluttonous and add harmful fat to our lives while starving our hearts and bank accounts.

Instead of feeling weighed down, the goal is to be lean and fit for the full life you were meant to live. Strive to be that thoroughbred in all areas of your life—more muscle and less fat.

Do Both at Once

This process doesn't stop. Patients start getting stronger—muscle tissue goes up, fat tissue goes down—and we tell them this is your goal for the rest of your life: more muscle and less fat. If we maintain that as a goal, we will be in great shape.

Most people we talk with are convinced they need to get the fat off first and then build muscle later. This simply won't work.

Apply yourself to doing both at the same time. In the same way, as you know by now, apply yourself to exercising your intellect, emotions, and spiritual life to build strength (muscle) in your whole person.

Often, those living the standard American lifestyle are not receiving the proper nutrition to optimize their genetic capacity to put on muscle. They're in a state of cellular starvation. Simply changing nutrition to take in the proper macronutrients (protein, carbohydrates, and fat) and micronutrients (antioxidants, vitamins, and minerals) will allow the body to build muscle, and burn fat with little or no exercise.

The body doesn't want to use muscle as fuel. That isn't how it was designed. The body wants to use fat as fuel. We want to get to a place where the body is using the fat that's coming in through our food and even burn some extra fat that's on our frame.

Once there is no excess fat on the frame, we always want to give our engines high-quality fuel to enjoy maximum performance and an energetic state of well-being.

Little by Little

A forty-year-old patient of ours was a good athlete and married to a physician. She was training for a big event, eating the standard American diet and feeling terrible. She worked out longer and harder but had stopped making gains.

She was not recovering, was tired all the time, and even found herself reaching for the anti-inflammatory pill bottle. Her body fat was probably 25 percent. She looked good on the outside, but after running so much, her baseline inflammatory markers and body composition were on the rise. She was alarmed to discover she was not as healthy on the inside as she had hoped. Looks can be deceiving.

We put her on an anti-inflammatory, muscle-building plan and adjusted her workout—actually telling her to work out a little bit *less*. She was over-training and wasn't getting results. Her poor nutrition would not support her exercise. She tried to exercise more to keep her weight under control, but that was a mistake. Over-exercise and poor diet were creating inflammation and making her sick.

In just three months, she felt much better, and her body fat went down to 13 percent. She was lean, happy, and full of energy. Her inflammatory markers returned to normal.

If she had not taken the time to be evaluated, five years down the road she may have been diabetic and faced the onset of heart disease. Yes, that is possible. Excess exercise, chronic inflammation, and hypercortisolism can lead to type 2 diabetes.

She recently told us, "I may be forty, but I will give anyone a run for their money. I feel unstoppable".

Little changes can create big results.

How Does Nutrition Help Burn Fat?

The calories burned with exercise certainly have some effect on body composition, but not nearly as much as people think. The vast majority of your return on investment in regard to positive body composition change lies squarely with your nutritional protocol.

Insulin plays a role in fat storage, thyroid function, stress hormone production, appetite, metabolism of cholesterol and triglycerides, and sleep. Optimizing insulin is the key.

Chronic production of insulin, predominantly occurring because of ingesting too much sugar, induces all cells, including muscle cells, to become insulin-resistant. When this occurs, the body begins to actually produce more insulin, mistakenly believing it needs more. Appetite increases, and the sleep cycle become dysfunctional. At this point, weight gain may begin, especially around the middle, progressing to metabolic syndrome and type 2 diabetes.

We can attribute this to the standard American diet, which is heavy in starches, sugars, grains, breads, and processed foods. Excess blood sugar with nowhere to go begins to get a grip on structural proteins in the body (AGEs, or advanced glycosylated end products), accelerating the aging process. Controlling insulin is the key.

You can control insulin to a great degree by what you put in your mouth.

Fat-Burning Foods
- non-starchy vegetables
- fruits
- healthy fats (avocados, nuts, and olive and coconut oils)
- organic or farm-raised protein

Fat-Storing Foods (avoid these)
- processed and fried foods
- soda
- sugars and artificial sweeteners
- MSG
- grains and breads
- corn
- soy

Keep in mind that your day-to-day health is massively influenced by your last meal of the day. Always make a point of making this a low insulin producing meal. Over time, your energy levels, sleep cycles, appetite, and body fat will normalize.

Download our Glycemic Index Food Chart and Muscle-Building Protocol in the book bonus section of our website. (See the back of the book for details on these and other bonus gifts to you.)

Time for PIES

Physically, your body was designed to be healthy, so it *wants* to get healthy. Give it the food and movement it craves and, little by little, you'll see improvement.

Intellectually, do you believe you can change how your body looks? You can. But you must first change how you look at your body. You might be hiding beneath an armor of excess fat, but the true you wants to emerge and enjoy life. Undercover the superhero inside you. You don't need a phone booth to change; you need to execute your plan.

Emotionally, when you read this chapter, what FRAUDS (fear, resentment, anger, unforgiveness, disappointment, and shame) did you feel? Are you willing to face these and become stronger? Have the courage to face them and overcome. This will build the emotional "muscle" you need to overcome the difficulties of life that try to throw you off course.

Spiritually, what can you do to care for your heart—to help your emotions and willpower? Consider listing affirmations that you can speak out loud daily. Here are a few:

1. I am always free of chronic stress and living a peaceful life.

2. I am in the process of removing excess fat and building more muscle.

3. I am successful in all my endeavors and make routine, high-quality decisions.

16

Hormones and Health

WE PUT THIS SECTION NEAR THE END, BUT NOT BECAUSE THE topic is not important. We put it here because it tends to be the "first response" in our society.

"Hormones can make your life better and your body lean" cry many ads from medical spas and men's clinics. However, hormones cannot override the standard American diet. They are important, but they cannot correct or overcome our bad behavior.

Hormones are substances produced by endocrine glands or organs that act on the body in many unique ways. Hormones can act inside cells in an *autocrine* manner. *Paracrine signaling* is a form of cell-cell communication in which a cell produces a hormone signal to induce changes in nearby cells, altering the behavior in those cells.

Endocrine signaling is where a gland secretes hormones directly into the blood to be carried toward distant target organs, where their actions are carried out. The major endocrine glands include the pineal gland, pituitary gland, pancreas, ovaries, testes, thyroid gland, parathyroid gland, hypothalamus, gastrointestinal tract, and adrenal glands.

In other words, hormones are one way the body is designed to fine tune itself to thrive. Hormone balance is essential for optimal health and well-being.

Like an automobile, our bodies need frequent tune-ups, periods of rest from the stresses of life, and—always—good fuel. What most people don't understand about hormones is that there is so much we can do with nutrition and lifestyle to keep our whole being running smoothly, and this includes optimization of hormones.

Examples of hormones include insulin (produced by the pancreas), thyroid hormone (produced by the thyroid), cortisol, epinephrine, norepinephrine (adrenal messengers), male and female sex hormones (produced by the testes and the ovaries), to name a few. Our internal chemistry balancing act occurs through signaling between the brain (hypothalamus and pituitary) and the end organs (thyroid, adrenals, male and female sex organs).

Insulin is unique in its response to blood sugar balance. Hormone balance is really a chemical version of a musical symphony going on inside our bodies all of the time. We do not need to be out of rhythm, which can often happen if we mistakenly target these hormones based on singular lab numbers. Our bodies have a good way of keeping hormones balanced. Medically speaking, this is called *homeostasis*. If lifestyle and nutrition become suboptimal, so do hormone levels. If hormone levels are out of balance, the effects that each hormone has on the system may be dampened.

Low thyroid equals increased body fat, cold body temperature, low mood, and dry hair and skin. Low adrenal hormones can lead to increased body fat, fatigue, and depression.

Low sex hormones can lead to increased body fat, low mood, low libido, and abnormal female and male function.

Insulin Overload

One of the biggest hormones of balance is insulin. Insulin is a hormone that manages blood sugar. Blood sugar can be toxic when levels get over 200, so our bodies have to keep sugar at a very controlled level all the time, and that's what insulin does.

Your brain basically says, "Blood sugar is getting a little high. Let's give it a little squirt of insulin."

Normally, when sugar levels get too high, warning buzzers sound to tell the body to reduce sugar. But with too much sugar intake over a period of time, the body becomes deaf to those signals and insulin levels go higher. This is the first stage of type 2 diabetes. And as we age, the receptors can get a bit rusty because of overstimulation. It's called receptor resistance, or insulin resistance.

If the cells cannot burn the sugar and put it into glycogen, it has to be taken out of the bloodstream—because it's toxic. But it has to go somewhere. So what happens? It's stored as fat. But at a certain point, the adipose (fat) cells in your body can no longer deal with the excess sugar. That's when you show up at the doctor with blood sugar over 200 and nothing can control it. Say hello to type 2 diabetes.

There is a lifespan on your pancreas. The pancreas is the endocrine organ that makes insulin. You can burn this organ out in thirty years with alcohol, lots of sugar, and standard American living. Or, it can perform perfectly to age one hundred.

Too much sugar and fat can also create abnormalities with the hormone leptin. This hormone is secreted by fat cells. It makes sense that leptin tells the brain when we have enough fuel (fat).

Leptin also tells the brain when the stomach is full. When we eat a lot, leptin signals the brain, "Hey, we're full down here, time to ask for the check!"

But the more fat cells you have, the more leptin you produce. And just like insulin resistance, you can become leptin-resistant.

Your body no longer hears the voice of appetite suppression, and you can guess how that works out.

All this creates the perfect storm for diabetes.

Check Engine

Put oil in the gas tank of your car and gas in the radiator, and you'll have problems. If your hormone system is frazzled—with all your buzzers buzzing and warning lights flashing—the cellular receptors can't detect the voice of a healthy, clean system. That's when the body goes downhill and drags the intellect, emotions, and heart along with it.

Fat makes estrogen and decreases the production of testosterone in both men and women. This drives down the body's ability to produce sex steroids because of weight issues. This is particularly troublesome because it can cause infertility issues.

When the body begins to shut down, the first system that often turns itself off is the reproductive system, because we can live without it. Your body will take energy from the reproductive system and try to shift it to another system.

When we stop eating all the inflammatory junk, hormones start to come into balance. Simply put, give the body what it needs and it will fix itself.

Before we prescribe hormones, we put the patient on a healthy living protocol for three months and monitor hormone levels. Putting a patient on hormones can become a lifelong sentence, because they can disrupt the body's natural regulators. Again, it's a matter of addressing the root causes rather than just applying a band-aid.

There's a lot of hype these days about the benefits of hormone supplements, particularly testosterone. If you have low sexual energy, low mood, or weight gain, it's common to be prescribed testosterone. It might give you more energy, but it's not always a real solution.

Men and women are losing testosterone faster than ever today. It goes right back to the obesity epidemic. As the fat tissue comes on, the fat tissue secretes leptin, which tells the brain that the body has plenty of energy stored. When the brain hears that, it's supposed to talk to the pituitary and the thyroid to say, "Let's crank up the metabolism—we need to burn this fuel!"

That's the way it *should* work: your body gets a little bit of fat and then burns it off. What is abnormal is the inundation of all these inflammatory foods that cause rapid fat gain. Instead of hearing that you have enough fuel, the brain hears that you have *no* fuel: "Hey, we're starving!" The brain talks to the pituitary and tells the thyroid to slow things down (which is exactly the opposite of a healthy reaction).

Still with Us?

Hormones 101 is a lot to take in, but here's the point: you can't expect to put the wrong fuel in your body and expect it to function well.

Just like your whole being (physical, intellectual, emotional, and spiritual) is designed to live in four-part harmony, your hormones are complex and interrelated. But they're also designed to help you get healthier when we cooperate.

If your medical professional has prescribed hormone treatment, don't stop the protocol. But do ask questions about what the end goal is.

Totally Tuned

There is a systematic way clean up the body, and it begins with lifestyle, which accounts for up to 90 percent of wellness.

Sometimes, if a patient's hormone (thyroid, male or female sex hormones) levels are alarmingly low, we'll use some medication, along with lifestyle changes, to save the system from the damaging effects of inflammation and dysfunction. We always go lifestyle first, neutraceutical/adaptogens second, then medications. This is a step-wise approach to treat hormone imbalance.

It's about *optimization,* which is not *normalization*—they are two different terms. Normalization is just getting something in a range based on the average population. Remember, comparing yourself to "normal" is not optimal, because America's *normal* is relatively unhealthy. Optimization is making you your best. Optimization is different for each person, since we're all unique individuals.

By now you've developed a healthy skepticism toward the word "normal." And with good reason. Normal people will die of heart disease. Normal doctors treat symptoms without addressing the root cause. It's normal to carry fear, resentment, anger, unforgiveness, disappointment, and stress.

But you have already decided to reject normal and live life to the fullest. You're not destined to chase around symptoms. With proper lifestyle, food, and rest, you can get better and better.

Menopause and Andropause

Menopause—and the male counterpart, andropause—conjures up all sorts of scary and foreboding symptoms. But don't resign yourself to worst-case scenarios.

Menopause is the decline in female hormones, usually beginning at age forty-five, plus or minus fifteen years. These hormones include progesterone, estrogen, testosterone, and DHEA. A woman's body is not *dependent* on them but *likes* each one of them for various reasons.

Estrogen has hundreds of functions in the body, including gut motility, cognition, cardiac markers, skin elasticity, bone health, moisturizing the eyes and mucous membranes, and more.

Progesterone is a neurosteroid and aids sleep and promotes the formation of the myelin sheath (protective coating of the nerves). It's a diuretic and is known as the *mother* hormone—at the top of the hormone "food chain," fed by cholesterol to become testosterone and estrogen. It can also be stolen to make the stress hormone cortisol. Often, because of its propensity to be stolen, progesterone will go down first as a result of a hyper-vigilant lifestyle and stress.

For females, menopause shows up with weight gain. They've had the same lifestyle for a long time, but all of a sudden things are different: they're tired, gaining weight, having trouble sleeping, anxious, and irritable. One day they are themselves, and the next day they are somebody else.

For some women, it starts ten or fifteen years before they stop having menstrual cycles. (The literal definition of *menopause* is the absence of menses, or menstrual cycles, for one year.)

For males, it's their wife who brings them to the clinic. And when men get there, they usually tell us they feel like they've lost their prime and can't exercise like they used too. When we ask if they're depressed, the answer is no.

Then we ask again. By the time we've asked the same question eight different ways, we finally hear the truth. "Well, I could go home and take a nap." So we ask if they are sleeping well, and usually they're having trouble sleeping.

Whether you're a man or a woman, know this: menopause and andropause are real—it's not just in your head.

If your symptoms are interfering with your life, you need a medical professional who understands all the forms of hormone therapy. You need somebody who knows the difference between bioidentical and synthetic hormone replacement.

Recent studies show that bioidentical hormones can create a decreased incidence of breast cancer and can be protective to the breasts, uterus, bones, and heart.

We had one particular fifty-two-year-old patient who told us he'd seen three different doctors about his symptoms. He was tired, his muscles were sore for days after he exercised, he was even a bit depressed. He had a general work-up, and the results were all normal.

He saw a rheumatologist at the recommendation of his primary doctor, who did a work-up for autoimmune disease and even infectious diseases, including Lyme disease. He also sought the help of an orthopedic physician. He had imaging studies and physical therapy and was placed on medications for soreness and pain, all to no avail.

Thousands of dollars later, he landed in our office. We ran our typical inflammatory/hormone panels on him and found him to have numerous inflammatory markers out of line, and his testosterone was in the mid-200s. (This level is well below optimal.) He was eating the standard American diet, had a few extra pounds of fat to loose, and led a very hypervigilant life.

We placed him on our anti-inflammatory nutritional plan, guided him through lifestyle modification to reduce stress, and started hormone replacement. Over a six-month period, his life rapidly turned around. With nutrition optimization, we were able to use the minimum amount of hormones to get the maximum result.

Of course, he had to do the work. We simply provided the right platform to launch a lifestyle of wellness.

This statement might ring a bell: *test, don't guess*. Putting this all together is super important. We know this has been a fairly technical chapter, but a basic understanding of your own body is crucial to making good choices.

Time for PIES

Physically, pay attention to your symptoms. Almost always, your body is trying to tell you what it needs to be well. If you are not listening, it will continue to talk louder until it gets your attention. Start to listen today. Don't let a heart attack, stroke, or other big event be the voice that must be heard before you pay attention. Bullheadedness is real, so don't be a hardhead. Listen!

Intellectually, our counsel is similar to above: don't rationalize or justify physical and emotional symptoms that take away from your quality of life. Respect yourself by taking note and seeking the counsel of a medical professional. Additionally, as we have routinely stated, evaluate how well your medical professional lives wellness in their own life.

Emotionally, take comfort in the fact that what you are experiencing may be related to hormones, and there is much you can do to "tune up" your body and mind. Rollercoaster emotions don't have to impact your self-esteem and spiritual life. Learn to simply breathe and relax. Your tune up may take a few months, but rest assured, you will start "running" better.

Spiritually, don't let physical and emotional symptoms take away your hope and vision for the future. With God's help, you can make wise choices to take care of all aspects of your being. Remember, God created you to experience health, love, joy, and peace.

17

Rediscovering the True You

WHETHER YOU SKIPPED OVER SOME CHAPTERS AND LANDED here or completed the book—welcome to the beginning! We know it might seem weird to say, *this is the beginning*, but it really is.

This moment can mark a turning point and a new beginning. You can become yourself—maybe for the first time in your life.

This is really the theme of this book, the theme of our clinic, and the theme of our calling in life: you were designed to enjoy life, and your entire being was designed to be well.

This book is not about becoming something you're not, it's about revealing the wonderful, God-given potential you were born with. And it's never too late to rediscover the true you.

The key to success is simple.

Take One Small Step Today

We've given you a lot of information and hopefully spark helpful introspection. It would be easy to become over with it all, but you don't have to.

We're just beginning. Take a deep breath. Congratulate yourself for investing in your future. Congratulate yourself for deciding to pursue wellness in all four areas of your life.

You've learned a bit about our stories and those of our wonderful patients. It's time to begin your own success story, right now.

Like most great tales with happy endings, the first scene might not be pretty or inspiring. You might be deep in wellness debt. You might feel trapped by bad habits and painful symptoms. But there is hope.

To take your first step, and the steps after that, you'll need heart. "Guard your heart above all else, for it determines the course of your life" (Proverbs 4:23 NLT). King Solomon wrote this proverb about three thousand years ago, but its wisdom is crucial for your journey. Physical wellness is important, but if you don't also guard your intellectual, emotional, and spiritual life, you'll fail.

This book is not a diet or a program, it's a lifestyle of loving yourself enough to make good choices. When you look in the mirror, choose to be happy with who you are and who you are becoming: the true you.

We want you to turn your whole life around. When you do, 'll be amazed at the momentum that's created and amazed at ⁺itive impact you'll make on your friends and family.

⁺ou "couldn't live without" become distant memories. ⁺ couldn't participate in become part of your ⁺ionships become vibrant and loving. It's all ⁺ to hear about those successes!

You Back

⁺ speak. If you are not careful, ⁺ere negativity and derogatory ⁺our mere existence a miserable

Day after day, year after year, you become what you think and speak. If most of the words that come out of your mouth have a negative tone to them, your life will move toward that negativity. Changing the process starts with evaluating your thoughts and how you speak. Every time you notice a negative thought, evaluate it and turn it around.

For example, if you normally think or say, "I am fat," change those words to "I am being weighed down with a coat of fat, but I am moving rapidly toward healthy body composition and optimum wellness." Speak this positive truth out loud, and invite your body, intellect, emotions, and spirit to the party.

The simple change in the attitude and action will help you get you to the gym and help you make better choices at mealtime.

We all want to experience a full, joyful life, right? Well, it doesn't start with running a marathon. It starts with a simple positive thought replacing a negative one. Every journey is one step at a time. Make the next step you take firm, positive, constructive, and uplifting. If you follow this simple walking lesson, you will make huge strides in life.

Face the FRAUDS

We all deal with FRAUDS—fear, resentment, anger, unforgiveness, disappointment, and shame. Part of caring for, and guarding, our hearts is facing these frauds.

Yes, we want you to go back and review the FRAUDS chapter, and all other chapters that stood out to you. (We said this was the beginning, remember?)

Reducing harmful cholesterol is good, but why stop there? Enjoy a better life by improving your relationship—with yourself, with God, and with those you love.

Endless Servings of PIES

Will you speak the following words out loud? It's a great first step.

"I was designed to live in four-part harmony—physically, intellectually, emotionally, and spiritually. My creator loves me, and I will love myself by taking care of all four facets of my being."

Say it one more time, please.

Welcome to your new beginning. Please don't think of this book as "finished." Keep it around as a reference and a reminder of hope. (And go back to the Setting Goals and Making Plans chapter to set your course.)

And please don't take this journey alone. Find a wellness professional (or contact us) who agrees with the principles of this book. Find a friend and an accountability partner to help you uphold your health goals.

And ask God for help and guidance along the way. He loves you and wants the best for every part of your life.

We love you too.
Mark and Michele

About the Authors

Michele Neil-Sherwood, DO

Michele L. Neil-Sherwood, Doctor of Osteopathy (DO), has had a successful private practice since 2002. She adopts a whole person approach, which is outcome-based and looks at each individual's unique needs.

Dr. Michele has been certified and trained through Cenegenics, BioTE Medical, Metagenics, Helm's Medical Institute, and AMMG and provides the following medical services: Age Management Medicine, Naturopathic and Functional Medicine, Lifestyle Coaching. She also provides soft tissue modalities of Osteopathic Manipulative Therapy and is certified in the Kettlebell Functional Movement Systems.

She has an extensive fitness and athletic background and lists the following achievements: Martial Arts (brown belt in judo and black belt in Tae Kwon Do), Strength Training/ Bodybuilding (multiple state and national titles), Russian Kettlebell System (RKC Certified, CK-FMS Certified, and Primal Move Certified) and Iyengar Yoga Methods.

Dr. Michele combines passion for wellness with compassion for people who want to improve the quality of their lives. She is a sought-out keynote speaker and presenter on various wellness and fitness topics.

Mark Sherwood, ND

Mark Sherwood, Naturopathic Doctor (ND), is the cofounder of the Functional Medical Institute in Tulsa, Oklahoma. Dr. Mark has been certified and trained in lifestyle modification and coaching, functional medicine, age management medicine, Nutrigenetics, as well as Translational Nutrigenomics.

Before embarking on his career as a naturopath, he was an Oklahoma state and regional bodybuilding champion, a professional baseball player, and a twenty-four-year veteran of the Tulsa Police Department, where he logged a decade of courageous service on the department's SWAT Team.

Mark's and his wife's activity DVDs and full line of nutritional supplements are the highest quality and are sold around the world. The couple cohosts a weekly television program airing on three networks.

Dr. Mark's passion for wellness motivated him to develop several wellness-based courses and presentations, which he teaches to law enforcement professionals, corporations, and churches throughout the United States and worldwide. He firmly believes that "each person has an awesome destiny and purpose in life, which can be revealed only through the pursuit of total wellness."

More Free Resources for Healthy Momentum

We couldn't possibly pack everything you need for yowur journey to wellness in one book. So we've created bonus resources for you.

Go to: www.SherwoodWellness.tv/bonus to sign up to receive our newsletter and unlock special resources and downloads.

See you there!

♪: FUNCTIONAL MEDICAL INSTITUTE

We founded the Functional Medical Institute to focus on complete healing, not disease management.
Our doctors and staff are dedicated to helping you stay healthy. We provide the knowledge, resources, and tools to give you a greater understanding of your health.

What is functional medicine?
Functional Medicine is a science-based medical practice that is patient-centered, not disease-centered. We incorporate the best diagnostic tools and technologies from conventional medicine, as well as emerging tests and tools to address the underlying root of the illness or disease.

We will help people all over the world:
- Gain muscle and optimize retention well into later years
- Lose fat and become a fat-burning engine
- Balance hormones using the latest hormone therapy
- Recover from, and prevent, injuries using PRP and Prolotherapy
- Discover your genetic blueprint which holds the key to nutritional, supplemental, and exercise prescription
- Develop a new relationship with food and food choices
- Regain and retain optimum health and highest quality of life

We spend time with our patients, get to know their story, understand their specific needs, and create a path for long-term health.

Contact us at the Functional Medical Institute
www.fmidr.com

CPSIA information can be obtained
at www.ICGtesting.com
Printed in the USA
LVHW02s2312080118
562330LV00004B/5/P